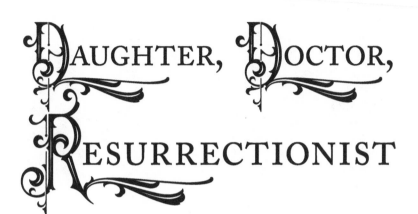

DAUGHTER, DOCTOR, RESURRECTIONIST

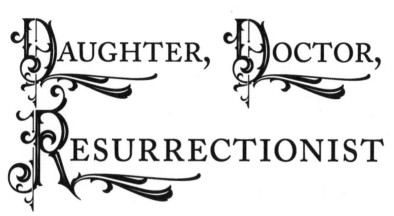

DAUGHTER, DOCTOR, RESURRECTIONIST

A True Story about
Medical Body Snatching
in 19th Century America

EDMUND MICHAEL VAN BUSKIRK

White River Press
Amherst, Massachusetts

Published by White River Press
PO Box 3561, Amherst, MA 01004
www.whiteriverpress.com

ISBN: 978-1-887043-52-6 hardcover
         978-1-887043-58-8 paperback
         978-1-887043-59-5 ebook

Copy Edit by Jean Stone, Falmouth, MA

Book and Cover Design by Douglas Lufkin
Lufkin Graphic Designs, Norwich, VT 05055
www.lufkingraphics.com

Library of Congress Cataloging-in-Publication Data

Names: Van Buskirk, E. Michael, author.
Title: Daughter, doctor, resurrectionist : a true story about medical body
    snatching in 19th century America / E. Michael Van Buskirk, MD.
Description: Amherst, Massachusetts : White River Press, 2020. | Includes
    bibliographical references.
Identifiers: LCCN 2019025712 (print) | LCCN 2019025713 (ebook) | ISBN
    9781887043526 (hardcover) | ISBN 9781887043588 (paperback) | ISBN
    9781887043595 (ebook)
Subjects: LCSH: Human dissection--Indiana--History--19th century. | Body
    snatching--Indiana--History--19th century.
Classification: LCC QM33.4 .V36 2020 (print) | LCC QM33.4 (ebook) | DDC
    611.009772--dc23
LC record available at https://lccn.loc.gov/2019025712
LC ebook record available at https://lccn.loc.gov/2019025713

Dedication

To Sarah

My daughter Sarah's exhaustive research in Ohio and Indiana made this book possible. Sarah's long hours searching, copying and transcribing smudgy newspaper articles, scratchy microfiche, musty court documents, and numerous obscure sources underlay the work's credence. Our 1994 interview with my father, and our research trips together in eastern Ohio, Cincinnati, and Fort Wayne stand among the fondest memories embedded in my 78-year-old sensorium. Sarah's legendary determination and her loving support sustained me to uncover and report the true story behind four generations of family lore.

Contents

Figures

Author's Note

All of the people, names, and events described herein are true, based upon historical records and contemporary newspaper accounts. On the other hand, some exact details, thoughts, and dialogue that transpired over a century ago could not be known in exactitude but were reproduced with closest adherence possible to the times and circumstances in order to stay true to the story revealed.

CHAPTER 1

The Squeamish Room

O N A COLD MORNING IN 1991, a handful of wan students, the first to arrive, pressed through the metal doors of the university anatomical laboratory. An unexpected silence and harsh overhead light accosted them. The smell, however, was as they had expected, caustic but tolerable, mitigated by the room's ventilation. They found their places around the assigned tables; heads moved in silence as eyes digested the surroundings.

Scrub sinks lined one of the mottled block walls; a green chalkboard extended the length of another. A lectern and a screen for displaying images from transparencies stood in front of the chalkboard. Glaring, caged, incandescent bulbs hung over ranks of two-dozen steel-topped tables whose surfaces tapered slightly toward a central hole positioned to allow liquid detritus to drip into floor drains below. Each table held a long, reeking mound beneath an oily shroud.

Aside from the electric lighting and indoor plumbing, the modern dissection laboratory of 1991 differed only in detail from those of earlier centuries. The oft-quoted *Memorials of John Flint South* described the 1813 dissection chamber of the famed London anatomist Sir Astley Cooper as "a squarish room lighted by two windows eastward and a square lantern in the ceiling . . . a large leaden sink under the windows was indiscriminately used for washing hands and washing subjects and discharging all the filth." South had referred to it as the "squarish" room, but, with repetition over time, it came to be called "squeamish" in both word and character.[1]

In preparatory lectures the day before, the professor had warned the medical students about the smells, the rows of bodies, and their own potential reactions to a supine corpse, that, in the coming months, would submit to their educational ministrations. The students had also been cautioned to examine carefully the face of their cadaver to ensure that it was a complete stranger. It had happened before (though not for many years) that students had recognized their corpse.

In the same prelude, the professor had spoken at length about the tradition in which they were about to become engaged. Anatomic dissection marked the beginning of all that would come for new physicians; yet, at the same time, it marked the end of a person's life. As the student doctors would learn to do with the living, they would struggle to balance their zeal for knowledge against their reverence for the body before them.

Until recently, dissection of the human cadaver had served as the threshold between the beginning student of medicine and an incipient doctor. It was by no means comparable to a mysterious initiation rite as if they were joining some secret society; rather, the obligatory and prolonged intimacy with the dead—with their vessels, their fibers, their viscera and excrement—would create an inescapable confrontation with human mortality that was destined either to bolster or undermine a student's resolve to become a physician. Cutting through the flesh of a fellow human being requires a certain sense of detachment that would serve them well in future, often unexpected, encounters with human frailty. Perhaps to gain a head start, medical students had long referred to their cadavers as "subjects."

---

1   Charles Lett Feltoe, M.A., *Memorials of John Flint South* (London: John Murray, Albemarle Street, 1884), 28–29.

The room quickly filled with freshly scrubbed students, most of them around 25 years old, all of them about to greet their first patients. They likely consoled themselves with the thought that these patients, at least, had already suffered their last pain; there was no risk of doing additional harm.

The professor entered the room; she smiled and nodded at her charges. At her instruction, the students retrieved green paper gowns and latex gloves from metal shelving, and then donned them in a parody of surgery. The garb, however, was for their protection, not for their subject's. Next, they gathered around their tables in groups of four, their hands swathed in latex, their work manuals and Gray's textbook of anatomy, 37th edition, open in front of them.[2]

At the lectern, the professor rapped on the microphone. "Ladies and gentlemen, you may begin. Today's dissection of the arm is outlined on the screen and begins on page four of your manual. Assistants will circulate through the room."

The four who stood around the first table tried to mask both their awe and their horror as they slowly drew back the oilcloth and revealed a naked, withered, dead old woman. As with the other subjects, she had been prepared in advance, injected with formalin, sometime before. A fine brass wire encircled one of her toes and held a tag that read: *1890–1990*. A hundred years of living, condensed to eight numbers and a dash; her stilled and shriveled hands had become twenty-seven small bones to locate and memorize. Under the students' tentative touch, the woman's body felt harder than they had expected—the skin was crinkled like an old salami. They had been taught to start their dissection with the skin of one arm, and then proceed to nerves and blood vessels, muscles and bones. One of the four, who had been elected by the others, readied himself to incise the dermis to the proper depth, sparing the deeper structures for lessons to come. A second

---

2   P.L. Williams, et al., *Gray's Anatomy*, 37th ed. (New York: Churchill Livingstone, 1989).

student read aloud from Gray's. The other two took notes, watched, and waited their turns.

As the students acclimated to the dead and the penetrating smells of formaldehyde that surrounded them, those who were not actively engaged in the dissection sometimes allowed their gaze to wander around the room to the cadavers being dissected on nearby tables—men and women, mostly old, some gaunt and weathered despite death and fixative. Others were obese: one bloated, beached carcass overhung the adjacent table's steel rim where the tentative students cut through great greasy layers of fat, heaving the globules into buckets on the floor. Those at the first table were glad that their corpse was thin.

The young dissector guided his new blade through the old woman's tough yellow skin. He admonished his colleague to steady the book that, over the coming weeks, would become progressively stained with oily remnants of their dissection. He peeled the shrunken dermis from the atrophied, chemically hardened muscles, trying to find fragile nerve strands within the mishmash of fat, tendons, vessels, and unidentifiable tissue. At first, it all appeared the same, but gradually, with careful work, yellow strands became the nerve plexuses as drawn in Gray's. Concentration upon the structures tended to suppress any consideration about the life that had ended for the old woman lying before him. She looked worn but somehow peaceful. Had the student let his mind drift from the intricacies of his work, he may have wondered (as he would wonder, in years to come, about real, living patients) how she had arrived on his watch. Some of the corpses in the room belonged to people who perhaps had outlived their families, their friends, and their resources, and ended up, unclaimed, on steel tables, succumbing to scalpels in uncertain hands. By 1991, many, if not most, cadavers had been donated through state-sponsored donor programs.

But the cold, shriveled body now lying before the young student had been born a century earlier, before automobiles, computers, or antibiotics. Her life, however, wasn't older than *Gray's Anatomy*: the classic text of gross anatomy written by Henry Gray was first published in 1858.[3] For over a century, Gray's had been the staple for beginning medical students to learn about the internal structures of the human body. Indeed, if any of the cadaveric subjects could have anticipated what would take place in that room well over a century later, it would have been that woman. Her hundred years of life provided lessons that could have taught them far more than the revelations of her anatomy. Though her memories were now quenched in formaldehyde, her life had been more intimately entwined with the process the dissectors were undertaking upon her body than any of them could have imagined.

Had they sought to learn more about the life of the cadaver being dissected, the students might have discovered that the woman had, in life, been one of two daughters of Aaron Elliott and Mary Jane Van Buskirk of Fort Wayne, Indiana. Her father had been a prominent doctor and a professor of surgical anatomy at the Fort Wayne College of Medicine. His obituaries described him as a much-admired physician and did not exaggerate when they said that he had had a hard life. His colleagues remembered him as a kindly man in a tall black hat who tended sick children even as his own four children were dying at home. They also undoubtedly recalled, but chose not to eulogize, the scandal that had rocked his life and scarred his early career in 1877, a scandal that had focused a spotlight on the practice of snatching bodies from fresh graves in order to supply cadavers to medical schools—cadavers just like the old woman's, and like all of the others, in that room on that day in 1991.

The scandal had preoccupied Aaron Elliott's youngest daughter, Bessie. In 1976, in her 86th year of life, she'd insisted that the bells had been rung in the courthouse to proclaim her father's innocence.

---

3   Henry Gray, *Anatomy: Descriptive and Surgical* (London: John W. Parker and Son, 1858).

"He never did it!" she cried, but then added, contradictorily, "After all, how were the students to learn?"

By that year, I, too, was a doctor of medicine. My own acquaintance with cadavers had begun in Boston, Massachusetts, on a September day in 1964. It was a Friday, and we were registering for classes that would begin the following Monday. We completed some paperwork and underwent a cursory physical examination of our eyes, ears, heart, and lungs. Only later, did they test our "intestinal fortitude."

We were assigned to groups of four and were sent outdoors and down a campus back alley to a windowless shed that was as ramshackle as an old chicken coop. A junior anatomy instructor garbed in a soiled white lab coat beckoned us from its doorway. Inside, my eyes soon adjusted to the dark interior and noticed a thick layer of sawdust carpeting the floor. Then I saw that along one wall, eerily illuminated from the sunlit doorway, deep shelves that held neatly stacked corpses, each frozen as hard as a forgotten ham in a basement freezer. A slimy yellow oilcloth clung to each body.

The instructor pointed to the nearest corpse, and the four of us, two on each end, lifted our cadaver and carried it outside, into the bright light of the warm fall day. Struggling under its literal dead weight, we moved back up the alley and traversed a small grassy area before re-entering the college building. We traipsed through a canteen where vending machines dispensed snacks, sandwiches, and drinks; we passed a few blasé upperclassmen casually chomping on sandwiches while our frozen corpses paraded before them. The four of us, who would become well acquainted as we slowly dismembered our burden in the coming months, crossed a narrow hall, marched up some stairs, and finally arrived at the anatomical laboratory. We placed the cadaver on the indelible scum of a stainless steel table so the body could defrost and drip over the weekend. (I never did understand why the cadavers had been frozen as well as fixed in formaldehyde. Perhaps it was to preserve the contents of body cavities like urine and feces, or perhaps simply to temper the foul smelling vapors or to facilitate storage and transport.)

By the following Monday morning, we found our cadavers were well defrosted and awaiting our first ministrations. Aside from our preliminary retrieval of the cadavers, my experience in the anatomy laboratory did not differ much from that of my physician-nephew who recounted to me his own experiences at Indiana University years later, at about the same time that Bessie's body lay on the dissection table.

Curiously, our experiences differed little from those of Bessie's father, A.E. Van Buskirk, in Cincinnati, Ohio, in 1875, or from those of my grandfather in Fort Wayne, Indiana, in 1902, or from my father's in Indianapolis in 1932. My father often recalled that one of his dissection partners would stuff a plug of tobacco in his cheek to stifle the slippery odor of formalin that never quite washes off.

CHAPTER 2

Inside the Body

I N BESSIE'S APPARENT NEED FOR CLOSURE to what had been her family's sentinel event, she had asked a pertinent, if rhetorical, question: "How were the students to learn?"

That question remains no small matter today, invoking more and more controversy as ethicists and lawmakers raise uncomfortable questions about the sanctity, the privacy, and the authority over a person's own body, unclaimed or not. Meanwhile, burgeoning fields of molecular biology, neurobiology, and genetics clamor for more space in every medical school curriculum.

By the end of the twentieth century, many medical academics had submitted that the time had come for gross anatomy—the study and firsthand dissection of all visible structures of the human body—to retreat from the center stage. The teachers of medicine from ancient times to the present day have grappled with the complexity of instilling in their students the necessary knowledge, skill, and practical experience to become physicians without compromising the standards of propriety and of care for those they are committed to help. Two decades before Bessie was born, when the events that haunted her century-long life had taken place, medical colleges were measured primarily by the quality and quantity of anatomical dissections that they could provide for their students. Microbiology and physiological chemistry were still in their infancy; dissection of cadavers, freshly unearthed from local cemeteries, was the core laboratory experience of academic medical education.

Even as a young girl, Bessie had understood the importance that human dissection held for medical students—both as the practical means to learn the intricate details of the human body and as the beginning of their passage toward becoming a physician. The topic weighed on her mind well until her ninth decade when she wrote to her nephew to explain that her father's students had needed to know about the "inside of the body" in order to become good doctors.

Like the Roman anatomist Galen, two thousand years before him, A.E. Van Buskirk had told his students that they needed to see and touch the structures themselves, not just read about them in books. Also, the most prominent early ninetieth-century surgeon and anatomist, Sir Astley Cooper, had exhorted his students and colleagues in 1823:

> You should know the nature of the human machine well, or how can you pretend to repair it? If you have a watch injured, you will not give it to a tinker to repair—you will get the best watchmaker you can to set it right. How, then can it be supposed that the finest and most perfect organization we know of, when out of order, should be consigned to the hands of unlearned persons?[4]

In the interim of two centuries, the intimate details of that most perfect organization—the human body—have subdivided its discernible parts to the multitude of the very atoms of its constitution. Similarly, the challenge for the contemporary medical student to understand the body's truly complete organization has been expanded by several orders of magnitude.

---

4 Sir Astley Cooper, *The Lancet*, Vol. 1 (Surgical Lecture, 1824), 1–8. Note that this was the first volume printed of this oldest and, even today, one of the most respected medical journals of Great Britain.

Bessie remembered tagging along with her father as he walked to his Saturday lectures at the medical college, his long black coat flapping in the wind behind him, as if to cloak the secrets of his past. By the turn of the century, he had largely overcome the stigma of his body-snatching scandal to become a successful, if somber, Fort Wayne physician. He was again teaching didactic and practical anatomy at the local medical school, now renamed the Fort Wayne College of Medicine. His students dissected cadavers that no longer had been stolen from the local graveyard, but had been legally acquired from the masses of bodies destined for the potter's field, unclaimed by family or friends.

For centuries, dissection of the human body served as a watershed over which fledgling medical students would learn to balance their natural reluctance to violate the human corpus against their compulsion to learn everything possible about its structure. Even as recently as 2002, displaced medical students in war-torn Afghanistan were so desperate to learn anatomy that they resorted to digging up the bodies of their own relatives.[5] The most dedicated medical students must temper their educational zeal against an innate abhorrence for touching, let alone dismembering, a human corpse. (*Note:* I have never forgotten how shocked and appalled I'd felt while on a tour of a prospective medical school when I happened to glance into a darkened corner of the anatomy laboratory only to see a garbage can overflowing with the remains of seemingly casually discarded human arms.)

Reverence for the dead runs deep in the human core as an acknowledgement of a life's end and the passage from one state to another, shrouded in corporal mystery and religious aura. Nearly every human society ritualizes disposition of their dead. The ancient Hebrews wrote: "He that toucheth the dead body of any man shall be unclean for seven days."[6] Pharaonic Egyptian embalmers

---

5   "Medical Schools Show First Signs of Healing from Taliban Abuse," *New York Times*, Jan. 15, 2002, A12.

6   Num. 19:11–22 (King James Version).

paradoxically were required to preserve, but were forbidden to violate, the dead body. They solved their dilemma by hiring urchin cutters who would make the incision into the corpse to receive the embalming fluid, and would then be obliged to bolt from the scene, as they were stoned by the priests to mollify the offended gods.[7]

Thus, for the new student of anatomy, the cutting, mutilating, holding, and discarding the parts of the human body might pose a profound revulsion, perhaps best expressed by Leonardo da Vinci:

> But though possessed of an interest in the subject, you may perhaps be deterred by natural repugnancy, or, if this does not restrain you, then perhaps by fear of passing the night hours in the company of those corpses, quartered and flayed and horrible to behold.[8]

The roots of academic anatomical study surely extended deep into the battlefields of prehistory, but they were formally sprouted among the ancient Greeks. Human dissection first blossomed during the third century BCE in the academic centers of Ptolemaic Alexandria where, for the first time and only time for another millennium, human anatomy became a legitimate, even desirable, subject of study for students of medicine. Herophilus of Chalcedon and Erasistratus of Ceos were the leading medical teachers in Alexandria. Both dissected human bodies, specifically, of executed criminals. Their influence extended, centuries later, to Rome, but Roman law prohibited human dissection, so the Roman anatomists resorted to animals. Dissection of human cadavers would not take place again for more than a thousand years until the dawn of the Middle Ages in Europe.

At the age of 32, the anatomist Galen (of the ancient Greek city of Pergamon, now a city in Turkey), who had studied in Alexandria

---

7   John H. Taylor, *Death and the Afterlife in Ancient Egypt* (Chicago: The University of Chicago Press, 2001), 54.

8   Sherwin B. Nuland, *Leonardo da Vinci* (New York, NY: Viking, Penguin Putnam Inc., 2000), 26.

from 152 to 157 AD, migrated to Rome where he served as physician to Emperor Marcus Aurelius. Galen performed public dissections, but of animals (monkey and dog), not of humans. He was mainly a follower of the teachings of Herophilus and disputed some of the concepts of Erasistratus as taught by his elderly rival, Martialius. When Martialius asked Galen which school of anatomists he followed, Galen replied that he chose what was good from them all, that to call any man a master was the mark of a slave. Galen never witnessed the dissection of a human body, but he drew his formidable insights from monkeys; he first drowned them in order to preserve their structures. Unlike his predecessors, colleagues, and successors, Galen performed the complete dissection himself, enabling him to make direct observations that might have been missed by others. Galen published many works on anatomy and physiology, concentrating his personal energy, productivity, and passion to reveal all the secrets of the nature of man. Eventually, Galen left such impenetrable influence upon his own society that the legacy of his dogma became virtually canonized for more than a thousand years.

As Rome crumbled under the onslaught of the northern European invaders, the centers of learning shifted east to Alexandria, Athens, Constantinople, and Baghdad. Eastern scholars recorded, translated, copied, and summarized the works of Galen into Greek, Syrian, and Arabic languages. Scholarly academic medicine became, for the most part, the philosophical learning, translating, and contemplation of Galen.

By 1050 AD, the Monastery of Monte Cassino, near Salerno, Italy, housed a large Christian hospital where the Monk Constantine the African reintroduced Galenic medicine back into the western world by retranslating the Arabic into Latin. By 1250, practical demonstrations of animal anatomy were again held on the Italian peninsula, using Galen's work as the sanctified text. Records of human autopsies also began to appear in Italy, but these were conducted to determine the cause of death in suspected murder cases, not for scientific inquiry. However, over the next century, the law in some Italian cities began to include provisions that mandated public dissection of the bodies of executed criminals. Such laws, in part, satisfied the needs for teaching human anatomy and simultaneously served as warnings to anyone who might have contemplated committing a crime that would be punishable by execution.

Mondino de Luzzi, known as the Restorer of Anatomy (1270–1326), performed public dissections of human bodies at Bologna in 1306. In the hot Italian climate, circumstances required that dissection be done quickly to minimize putrefaction of the body. The dissection was completed, not in logical anatomical order, but in the order of the susceptibility of tissue to decay, beginning with the internal abdominal organs, then the chest, the head, and, finally, the extremities.

Soon, many European universities offered their students instructional demonstrations of Galenic anatomy. Perched upon a dais far above both the students and the cadaver, the august professor would drone from the Galenic text, well out of range of the vile stench emanating from the anatomical subject below. As the professor described the important structures, a junior assistant would languidly point to them while using a wand often several feet in length to maintain a healthy distance from the foul body. A demonstrator barber-surgeon performed the actual dissection on the putrefying body, plowing his knife indiscriminately through critical structures, and then tossing loose scraps of flesh to stray dogs that lurked beneath the table. (*See Fig. 1.*)

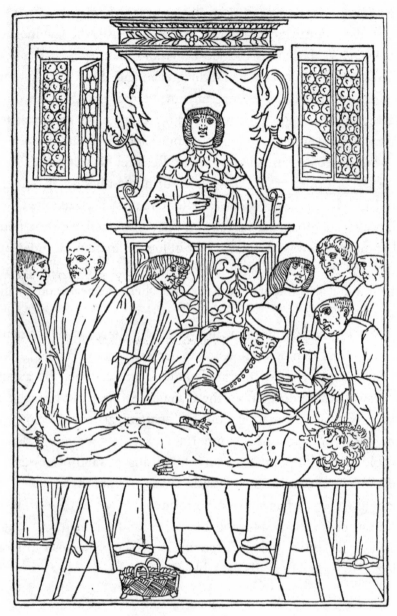

Figure 1. Anatomic dissection in fifteenth-century Italy, showing the professor high on his dais, reading from Galen; his assistant (far right) points to the cadaver while the "menial demonstrator" dissects. From Mondino de Luzzi, frontpiece of Mondino's Anothomia.[9]

---

9   Charles Singer, *The Evolution of Anatomy* (New York, NY: Alfred A. Knopf, 1926), 77.

Laws permitting a requirement for human dissection were passed in Europe during the fourteenth century. In 1387, the University of Florence was, by law, to be provided three bodies of "alien criminals" each year for dissection. To preserve the utility of their body, it was stipulated that these condemned individuals were to be hanged, not burned or beheaded. An anatomy student at the university was selected to make the arrangements for a room where the dissection would take place. Other cities and universities throughout Europe soon followed suit, providing for public dissections to be held at least once yearly.

Knowledge of anatomy had become essential not only to physicians but also to artists who were interested in the most accurate depictions of the human body. Leonardo da Vinci became an accomplished, self-taught anatomist in his own right. At first, Michelangelo was so repulsed by the process that he eschewed dissection, but he ultimately realized its importance to his work and returned to anatomy with unmitigated vigor. The Italian artist, Bartholomaus Torre of Arezzo, kept cadavers or their parts in his rooms for ready reference. His assiduous study amid the putrefying flesh was reputed to have led to his premature demise at age 25.[10]

By the sixteenth century, anatomic instruction had become an accepted part of the university curriculum in Europe, but the work of Galen remained the inviolate canon. The leading anatomy professor of France, Jacobus Sylvius, held the work of Galen to be divine, and thus inviolate, but one of his students, Andreus Vesalius, grew impatient with his professor's dogma. He grabbed the instruments from the barber-surgeon to complete detailed examinations himself. As Vesalius began to record consistent differences between the human anatomy that he observed and the anatomic descriptions that he read in Galen, he grew to doubt the legitimacy of some of the Galenic canon.

---

10 James Moores Ball, *The Body Snatchers*, repr. (New York, NY: Dorset Press, 1989), 25. First published 1928.

Much has been made of Vesalius's courage to break with the dogma of Galen, for which he was castigated by his contemporaries, but he was too rigorous a student to deny the evidence of his own eyes. Vesalius was so driven to make direct observations that he frequented the graveyards of Montfaucon and the Cemetery of the Innocents. Bodies of all the executed criminals in Paris were brought to Montfaucon, where the corpses were hung from beams until they were reduced to their skeletons. However, when Vesalius reached them first, he took the bodies down and dissected them, often fighting off stray dogs in the process. In 1543, he published his classic work, *De Humani Corporis Fabrica*, which set the stage for the crucial role of firsthand dissection of fresh cadavers in the teaching of medicine for centuries to come.[11]

---

11 J.B. deC.M. Saunders and Charles D. O'Malley, *The Illustrations from the Works of Andreas Vesalius of Brussels* (Cleveland, OH: World Publishing Co., 1950).

CHAPTER 3

The Demonstrator

IN TIME FOR THE FALL TERM OF 1877, Doctor Aaron Elliott Van Buskirk, barely 30 years old, arrived with his new bride, Mary Jane (Gray), at Fort Wayne, Indiana, to assume his position as demonstrator of anatomy at the as yet unproven college of medicine. He hoped to soon be promoted to professor.

A.E. had always wanted to be a doctor. He remembered stories about his aunt, Dr. Anne Elizabeth Van Buskirk, who, though lacking formal medical training, had been one of the first women doctors in rural Ohio. In the same vein, the ordeal of his father's protracted illness and death had seared a resolution to become a physician into his youthful mind.

Descended from the earliest settlers of Dutch colonial New Netherlands and of the post-Revolutionary War migration to the western territories, Aaron Elliott Van Buskirk was born to Jacob and Mary Ann Van Buskirk on September 27, 1847, at Harrisburg, Carroll County, Ohio.[12] Their families had settled in the valley of the Tuscarawas River, not far from the Pennsylvania border. Aaron's family, however, soon moved west to Indiana, and then to Mercer County, Illinois, on the Mississippi River, where his father died, presumably of malaria on September 24, 1857.

---

12 Van Buskirk, E.M. *The Van Buskirks of Indiana* (Amherst, MA: Genealogy House, 2018).

After ten years of arduous and migratory marriage, Jacob Van
Buskirk had left Mary Ann widowed on the eastern bank of the
Mississippi with four young children including an infant, Mary
Belle. Life had taken a difficult turn for Mary Ann Elliott Van
Buskirk, who could do nothing but return home to her family in
Ohio. As she stood on the platform at the railroad depot carrying
little Mary Belle, with ten-year-old Aaron holding the hands of
his brothers, John and Joe, Mary Ann must have wondered what
lay in store for them. The young widow did manage to move her
entire family back to Ohio, where Aaron was bound out to the
nearby farm of an uncle, most likely Mary Ann's brother. When
he turned 18, Aaron moved back to Monroeville, Indiana, near
his uncle James Van Buskirk who had sixteen children on their
family farm. The two oldest children, George and Joseph, had
fought in the Civil War. George was killed at Gettysburg, but
Joseph returned to Monroeville in 1863. A.E. greatly admired his
older cousin, Joseph, who inspired and encouraged A.E.'s similar
ambitions to become a physician.

Like many of the doctors of that time, the cousins Joseph and
A.E. Van Buskirk acquired their medical training in bits and pieces,
working, farming, and teaching school in the interims. Most likely,
Joseph "studied" with a local practitioner or preceptor in Wisconsin
before receiving a degree in medicine from a local college there. A.E.
later joined Joseph in Wisconsin, perhaps to help maintain Joseph's
farm while the elder cousin completed his education. By 1872, after a
brief teaching stint in central Iowa, A.E. returned to Ohio to obtain
his own medical credentials by working for a practicing physician. In
reality, such preceptorships with practicing physicians often provided
more cheap labor to the senior doctor than any formal education
for the apprentice. A country doctor may have owned one or two
medical books and perhaps a few essential instruments. Mostly,
they needed assistants to maintain their herb and root garden, grind
medications in their pharmacy, and help with difficult obstetrical and
fracture cases. Occasionally the two, preceptor and aspirant, would

retrieve one of their failures from the local graveyard to advance their anatomical knowledge. Despite its academic shortcomings, the preceptorship was the sort of on-the-job training that was sufficient for an entrepreneurial young doctor to obtain a medical license and to launch a career.

In the post-Civil War period, it was possible to obtain medical training and licensure by several means: on-the-job training, taking a few classes at the local college, or taking a full course to receive a doctor of medicine academic degree from a recognized college of medicine. Many physicians tried all three routes, often starting with a preceptorship and later attending a college of medicine. In actual practice, it probably didn't really matter much because medicine was practiced indiscriminately on the basis of century-old beliefs about humors and phlogistic forces within the ailing body. Each of the various categories of doctors, from the so-called "regulars" through the homeopathic, Thomsonian, naturopathic, eclectic, and hydrotherapeutic practitioners, experienced about the same dismal degree of success. Of course, even today, the majority of illnesses that people encounter—common colds, muscle strains, and minor infections—usually, but not always, resolve through their own natural course, a resolution for which some practitioners are only too happy to claim credit.

By the late 1830s, public frustration with doctors' incompetence, bickering among the many factions of medicine, and the rise of Jacksonian populism induced many state legislatures throughout America to repeal most, if not all, regulations governing the licensure of doctors. But after the Civil War, the European advances in the science of medicine began to be felt in North America. The states again began to develop new regulations that would govern the medical practice, and they established new guidelines for education and licensure of physicians. Although many physicians held licenses based on their practical experience, by the 1870s, it was advantageous to a young physician to have a medical degree granted by an officially chartered college of medicine.

The medical training of A.E. and Joseph Van Buskirk overlapped and intersected, A.E. always a few steps behind his older cousin, as each struggled to gain an education and maintain a livelihood. For a short time after the war, Joseph Van Buskirk farmed, ran a sawmill business, and taught school in Monroeville, Indiana, where A.E. later succeeded him. Then, A.E. joined him in Wisconsin, perhaps to maintain his farm while the elder cousin completed his medical education. Ultimately, they parted ways. Joseph moved west to the Black Hills of South Dakota where he practiced medicine and ran a drug store. By 1872, after a brief teaching stint in central Iowa, A.E. had returned to Ohio to obtain his own medical credentials.

A.E. Van Buskirk settled and taught at the local grammar school in Millersburg, Holmes County, Ohio, where his aunt had lived after her marriage. In Millersburg, A.E. met Mary Jane Gray, who was 24 years of age in 1872 and the daughter of a local scion, Robert Gray, who farmed, had a plastering business, and served as president of the Holmes County Agricultural Society. The Grays were among Millersburg's more prominent families.

In addition to enjoying the society of Mary Jane Gray, A.E. was fortunate to meet the most respected physician in Millersburg, Dr. Joel Pomerene, who agreed to precept him. Dr. Pomerene had learned his doctoring at the side of a local Holmes County practitioner before the Civil War, but like many young physicians of his time, he wanted the credibility and knowledge implicit in obtaining a full medical degree. He enrolled at Jefferson Medical College of Philadelphia and graduated in 1858. After the war, Pomerene maintained a well-known practice in Millersburg on Main Street, opposite the county courthouse. (The community hospital now bears his name.) Dr. Pomerene also became one of the first faculty members in the Medical Department of Wooster College. Wooster was about an 18-mile ride north of Millersburg, but the medical department was located in Cleveland. In 1874, A.E. enrolled in the Wooster Medical Department for one year, with Dr. Pomerene as his faculty preceptor.

After the apprenticeship with Dr. Pomerene and the course at Wooster, A.E. qualified for a license to practice medicine. In 1875, he returned to Monroeville, Indiana, where he established his first medical practice. Like most young country doctors struggling to survive, he taught in the same local high school where his education had begun ten years earlier. He bought a small house adjacent to the schoolhouse and near the railroad depot. The small rural town of Monroeville probably supported the farmer-doctor from Ohio, and he seemed to be settling well into his life: he had fulfilled his dream of becoming a doctor, lived among his extended family in Monroeville, and was setting out on a successful, if pastoral, life.

But, settling in was not to be. First, the eligible Mary Jane Gray was still in Millersburg, and A.E. needed to make clearer plans for a future with her. The apprentice-trained doctor-farmer-schoolteacher in Indiana, however, might not have had sufficient prospects to encourage the Grays of Millersburg to approve the family union. At the same time, some of the physicians in Fort Wayne, the county seat and second largest city in Indiana, had grandiose plans for a regional college of medicine. There was already a large, well-respected medical community with an active local medical society. While many of the Fort Wayne town physicians worried about competition and bickered among themselves, the smaller surrounding rural communities desperately needed knowledgeable doctors. The few physicians who drifted west from the eastern cities were neither sufficient in number nor competence to fill the need. Over the opposition of a few outspoken colleagues, a circle of Fort Wayne doctors, with the backing of Fort Wayne's leading citizens, advanced the development of a local medical college. Knowing that A.E. Van Buskirk was part of a local family and had recently obtained his certification, they probably approached him about becoming one of the founding faculty. A.E. jumped at the chance but, like his mentor, Dr. Pomerene, he wanted to complete his training with a full-fledged degree in medicine. Thus, he closed the doors of his practice in Monroeville, but kept his license and

his home. In the fall of 1875, he matriculated in Cincinnati at the
Medical College of Ohio. (*See Fig. 2.*)

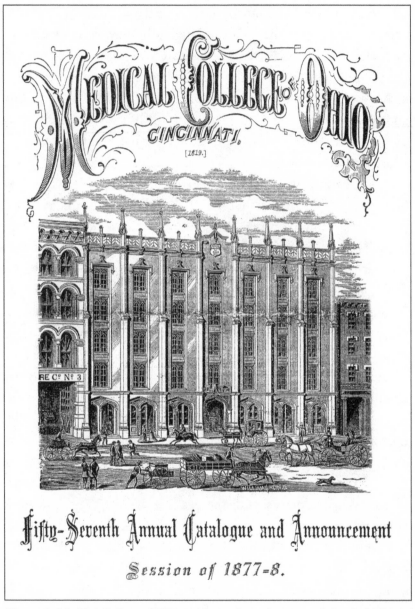

*Figure 2. Medical College of Ohio as depicted on the cover of the 57th Annual
Catalogue and Announcement.*

CHAPTER 4

A College of Medicine

N MARCH 14, 1876, while A.E. Van Buskirk was studying in Ohio, Christian Stemen and Harold Clark disembarked at the Fort Wayne railroad depot from the afternoon train from Cincinnati and walked the ten city blocks down South Calhoun Street to the Aveline Hotel. (*See Fig. 3.*) On their way into the lobby, the men passed Ayer's Drug Store on the first floor. Ignoring the evening *Sentinel* on display at the newsstand and the staccato of colliding ivory emanating from Kelly's billiard room, the men ascended the grand central stairway to a second floor salon. Cigar smoke wafted about the gas wall sconces as they waited for their Fort Wayne colleagues to join them. The plan was to convene in order to work out the final details of a proposal they'd been debating for months. Stemen, Clark, and their colleagues were doctors; they were discussing the potential of founding a local medical college.

The venerable Dr. Benjamin Studley Woodworth had called the meeting, but it was more than a medical matter. Some powerful local business scions had been urging the establishment of such a college. These gentlemen included Hugh McCulloch, the politician who was secretary of the treasury under presidents Lincoln and Andrew Johnson, and, by then, was president of the State Bank of Indiana; and Joseph K. Edgerton, president of a local railroad. The

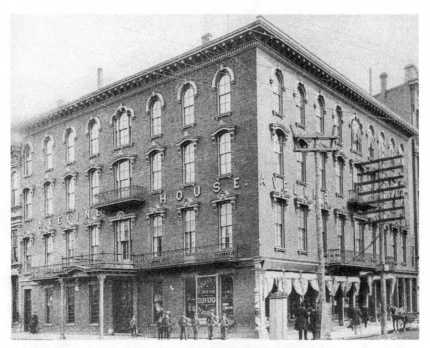

Figure 3. Aveline House Hotel, ca. 1889, Fort Wayne, Indiana. Reproduced with the permission of the Allen County-Fort Wayne Historical Society.

social, political, and business leaders saw a medical college as an enhancement of their growing community, one that would bring new intellect, new business, and new credibility to Fort Wayne. In their eyes, it would reinforce Fort Wayne's claim to be a full-fledged city that was comparable to Indianapolis and Cincinnati, both of which boasted medical colleges. At the same time, they hoped the new enterprise would assure a steady supply of new doctors for their growing community.

Three other businessmen—A.C. Remmel, whose building on Broadway and Washington would become the first site of the fledgling school; John Bass of the huge Bass Foundry and Machine Company; and Col. R.S. Robertson, Medal of Honor hero and local entrepreneur—rounded out the business representatives at the Aveline. These school founders had worked out their differences in the preceding months and were there to imprint the finishing touches on the school documents. They agreed to establish a new medical college to be known as the Medical College of Fort Wayne. McCulloch, Edgerton, Bass, and I.D.G. Nelson (president of Lindenwood Cemetery), would sit on its initial board of directors to assure its smooth launch.

Among the most interesting of the original founders was Dr. Christian Stemen, then of Cincinnati. Although he had the least experience with the affairs of medical schools, Stemen would ultimately rise to the greatest prominence. Like many fledgling doctors, he had begun teaching grammar school while attending medical classes, in his case at the Eclectic Medical Institute of Cincinnati, from which he graduated in 1864. "Eclecticism" was one of the new "cults" of medicine—along with Thomsonian medicine, botanico-medicine, physio-medicine, and homeopathy—which, after the Civil War, had made substantial inroads into the practice and credibility of the old-time regular or "allopathic" physicians. Since one system was about as effective, or ineffective, as another, aspiring doctors sometimes tried one first, later another. Stemen was restless by temperament, sliding readily from one role to another. He also became a licensed preacher in the United Brethren Church and preached from the Sunday pulpit for most of his life. By the 1870s, Stemen had decided to pursue, in addition to his "eclectic" certificate, a regular medical degree from the Medical College of Ohio. He graduated in 1875. Stemen wrote the definitive textbook on railway surgery, which was based on his experiences with the many injuries in the rail yards at Fort Wayne. He eventually became nationally prominent as a surgeon, as a trustee of Purdue University, and as a candidate for the United States Congress.

By contrast, Stemen's Cincinnatian colleague, Harold A. Clark, was a reclusive, sour sort of man, shrinking from conflict, which was an oddity in a day when many physicians were bombastic and confrontational. After graduating in 1869 from Starling Medical College in Columbus, Ohio, the predecessor to the Ohio State University School of Medicine, Clark served as physician to the Ohio Penitentiary until 1873, when he was appointed first, demonstrator, and later, professor, of chemistry at the Medical College of Ohio.

Among the local contingent, Benjamin Woodworth was the senior medical statesman, having been one of Fort Wayne's first physicians. It was natural that the Charles Wright family would choose him to care for the gravely ill Charles, but Dr. Woodworth was more than just a local doctor. He was imbued with a professional and academic fervor that set him apart from other young doctors and went beyond the mere craft of medicine. In 1846, when he set up his practice in Fort Wayne, Woodworth acknowledged that antebellum American medical care was barely improved from the practices of Hippocrates and Galen. He admitted that it offered little real benefit to patients. He decried the noxious methods of traditional medicine—the bleedings and the administering of horrific poisons designed to drive out internal imbalances and toxicity. He promoted the new scientific rationale that had taken hold in Europe and was gaining slow but inevitable credence after the American Civil War. For all his iconoclasm, Woodworth had establishment standing—he was past-president of the Indiana State Medical Society, respected among his colleagues and throughout his community for honesty and intellect. His leadership was crucial to the success of the new college, and he shared the businessmen's devotion to Fort Wayne's aspirations.

Just as Woodworth was regarded as the first physician in northeast Indiana, so his colleague across the table, William Herschel Myers, was regarded as the area's first surgeon. As surgeon to the 30th Regiment, Indiana Infantry in the early years of the Civil War, he sustained injuries in a horse-riding accident; his subsequent early discharge from military service would haunt him in the rancor of the professional battles to follow.

The founders held the official introduction of the new college on the Tuesday after the meeting at the Aveline Hotel; they invited the broad community of physicians, business leaders, and other interested parties. Colonel Robertson chaired the session, remarking that he was "honored to preside over a meeting of men whose object would be so beneficial to mankind." He presented the college, its enterprise, its corporate seal, its board of trustees, and its faculty of fourteen local and regional doctors.

Many of those present took a more jaundiced point of view than had the old colonel. They suspected that the motives were more base than a "benefit to mankind." It was apparent that the enthusiasm of the original group who had met at the Aveline was not universally shared by their medical colleagues. Certainly, the school had been developed as a proprietary business for its doctors and investors; such was the basis of virtually every medical college of the time. While the *Fort Wayne Daily News* extolled the virtues of the new school, the *Sentinel* depicted it as an "Esculapian Enterprise."[13] One doctor's anonymous letter to the *Sentinel*'s editor impugned the project as unnecessary and pecuniary, and characterized the principals as incompetent teachers of medicine. His rapier spared only "one old man," Benjamin Woodworth, who, the writer contended, was being drawn to a venture he did not completely understand. Woodworth defended himself as a willing and enthusiastic participant and asserted that the institution was necessary for the community. Another published letter to the editor drew extensively from William S. Edgar's editorials in the *St. Louis Medical and Surgical Journal* that broadly decried the multiplicity of non-credentialed diploma mill medical colleges in the West and castigated the avarice and ignorance of his medical colleagues.[14]

Local doctors who were excluded from the new endeavor, and who publicly opposed it, called for an immediate assembly of the county medical society to discuss the matter. Their meeting of March 21 passed a resolution that condemned the new college

---

13 "Esculapian Enterprise," *Fort Wayne Daily Sentinel*, March 15, 1876.
14 *St. Louis Medical and Surgical Journal*, 11 (September 1874): 485. William S. Edgar, ed.

of medicine and recommended that the program be abandoned. In the same vein, the *Kendallville Standard*, from about 25 miles north of Fort Wayne, expressed doubt about the professorial qualifications of the new faculty and asserted that it was primarily a financial venture on their part. In contrast, the Northeastern Indiana Medical Society, based in neighboring Angola, Indiana, a bit farther to the north, denounced the cynicism of the local critics and endorsed the new school as a source of needed medical practitioners. Some viewed training local young men as the most logical method to assure a reliable supply of doctors.

The Reconstruction era after the Civil War had become nearly revolutionary for the advances in clinical medicine, both conceptually and in practice. New ideas such as the germ theory, antisepsis, anesthesia, microscopy, anatomic pathology (autopsies), and modern surgery rendered the old practices of bleeding, purging, and poisoning obsolete. The new methods threatened the business of established doctors and, perhaps more crucially, their personal identity. During the Civil War, the ubiquitous administration of calomel—chloride of mercury—had caused so much misery among the union soldiers that the Surgeon General ultimately banned its use over the protestations of the older doctors.[15] The new recommendations for surgeons to wash their hands and change their cloaks before performing operations loomed as a virtual confession of responsibility for the postoperative infections that had haunted surgeons and killed their patients in the past. Some physicians embraced the new ideas as the foundation for better medicine. Others lamented the changes as they recoiled from their own ignorance.

Aside from these grander shifts and tensions, opposition to the new school was also a simple matter of professional competition. It was no accident that those physicians in the surrounding

---

15 George W. Adams, *Doctors in Blue* (Baton Rouge, LA: Louisiana State University Press, 1952).

communities who drew customers from a different population generally favored the school, while many Fort Wayne doctors opposed it. They feared that faculty members would acquire an instant professional stature that would serve them well in attracting patients, and that they would directly profit from their affiliation by requiring students to purchase tickets to attend their lectures—an entirely new source of income unavailable to those doctors who were not on faculty. Also, once students had graduated, they would no doubt gratefully refer difficult cases to their former professors.

By 1876, there were already four medical colleges in Indiana, with more to come. Perhaps most famous of the early Hoosier proprietary medical colleges was the Indiana Medical College of the Medical Department of La Porte University. The school was only open for five years, from 1844 to 1849, but it managed to graduate one William Worrall Mayo, whose sons founded the famous clinic bearing the family surname in Rochester, Minnesota.

Typically, as would prove the case in Fort Wayne, medical colleges were not affiliated with any parent university and were free to grant whatever academic, professorial titles they considered appropriate. Virtually every teacher became an instant "professor." Medical colleges imposed virtually no admission requirements upon prospective students beyond their ability to pay a modest matriculation charge and lecture fees that were levied directly by the individual faculty members who competed mightily for the attention of the matriculates. Even Harvard Medical School, acclaimed by some contemporary critics for its high standards, used local practitioners as faculty without regard to their academic qualifications. When some of the university-affiliated medical colleges attempted to improve standards and lengthen their curricula, they lost so many students that they returned to the established laxity. The Harvard medical faculty scoffed at the absurdity of President Eliot's proposal to require medical students to pass a written examination, because less than half of the class was able to write.[16,17]

Outside of the professional squabbles, the public was, at best, ambivalent toward a medical college in its midst. Most people viewed doctors as little more than scary charlatans, dispensers of those horrific poisons, virtual ambassadors to the grim reaper. They had no desire to see such talents incubated locally. Medical colleges were ghoulish, unclean places reeking of disease, decay, and death, from which exuded the very putrefying miasma that the old guard physicians had decried as the source of sickness. Not to mention the rumors that the opening of medical colleges in other communities had invariably led to bodies being stolen from local graveyards in order to supply the anatomic dissection laboratory.

Even before the medical college was established in Fort Wayne, some of the city's physicians had been accused of opening recently dug graves, pilfering the bodies, and shipping them to schools in Ohio and Michigan. In one case, a medical student from Fort Wayne recognized his recently deceased relative on the dissection table in Ohio. Thus, there already existed a regular traffic in newly deceased bodies, shipped throughout the Midwest to medical colleges who were in constant need of anatomic dissection material. For many Fort Wayne residents, the abstract notion of better and more available medical care was not sufficient to outweigh their more concrete and ominous expectations of a nefarious medical college in their midst.

Despite the opposition of the county medical society and an ambivalent public, the founders proceeded with their plans to open the Medical College of Fort Wayne in the fall of 1876 with Christian Stemen serving as its first dean. Harold Clark was named the professor of anatomy. They acquired space on the upper floors of A.C. Remmel's building on the corner of Broadway

16 Gerald L. Geison, ed., *Physiology in the American Context, 1850–1940* (New York, NY: Springer, 1987), 79–84.

17 Kenneth M. Ludmerer, *Learning to Heal* (New York, NY: Basic Books, Inc., 1985), 12.

and Washington, about a mile from the Aveline. (*See Fig. 4.*) The college rooms on the second story were deemed "commodious and convenient" in the college bulletin. The building also held an amphitheater that could seat several hundred students, far more than ever matriculated. It was also fitted with "chemical-physiological laboratories, anatomical dissection rooms and museums." It wasn't long before its Fort Wayne neighbors filed a complaint about the fetid stench arising from the building. Because behind those walls, a great deal was going on.

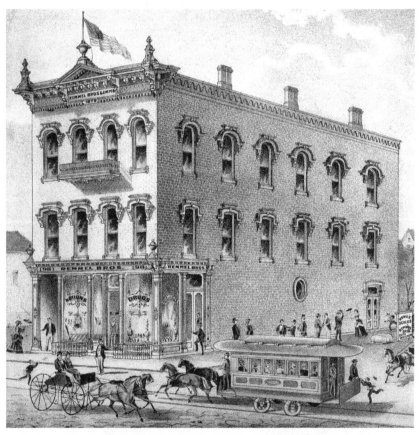

Figure 4. Remmel Building, Fort Wayne, Indiana. The first Medical College of Fort Wayne was housed on the top two floors with the entrance on the side at the rear of the building, as seen lower right in the etching. Reproduced with the permission of the Allen County-Fort Wayne Historical Society.

William Wright's drug store was on the first floor, facing Washington Street, and proved convenient for the college. Sympathetic physicians typically informed the pharmacist when one of their patients was near death. The pharmacist then called upon the anatomist who, in turn, arranged for the "resurrection" after the body's interment.

The new college had recruited an initial faculty of fourteen doctors, including its five founders: A medical curriculum that primarily consisted of didactic lectures required a substantial faculty to carry the load. No written curriculum remains from 1876, but it probably differed little from that of 1881. Students listened to lectures six days per week—from 9:00 a.m. until 5:00 p.m. on Tuesday, Wednesday, and Friday and until 3:00 p.m. on Saturday. After the morning lectures on Monday and Thursday, they attended afternoon clinics with various faculty physicians. The classes were generally one hour each with two hours for lunch.

The subjects covered were "Theory and Practice of Medicine," "Surgery and Clinical Surgery," "Pathology," "Obstetrics," "Anatomy, Descriptive and Surgical," "Materia Medica and Therapeutics," "Eye and Ear and Clinical Ophthalmology," "Physiology and Clinical Medicine," "Chemistry and Toxicology," and "Diseases of Children." Eleven textbooks were required with several options available in each subject, including the famous *Gray's Anatomy*, Austin Flint's *Textbook of Medicine*, and Samuel Gross's *System of Surgery*. Although the students had clinics only two half days per week, these included surgery, medicine, chest diseases, gynecology, pediatrics, urology, and eye and ear clinics.

By 1881, the brochure for the Medical College of Fort Wayne boasted that the school more than met the requirements of the Association of American Medical Colleges, a body that continues to monitor the quality of American institutions of medical education today. Students paid $5 to matriculate at the school, $40 for each professor's course, $5 for a professor's single lecture, $5 to the anatomy demonstrator for use of the dissection lab, $5 to the hospital, and $25 to graduate. Dissection of at least two cadavers, either at the school or elsewhere, was required for graduation.

Fifteen students completed the first class and graduated in February 1877. It was in August of that year that Aaron Elliott Van Buskirk, a young physician from Monroeville, recently graduated from the Medical College of Ohio, joined the faculty to assume the post of demonstrator of anatomy.

CHAPTER 5

The Season of Resurrection

HE MEDICAL COLLEGE OF FORT WAYNE opened for its second fall term in September 1877. The faculty and students entered through a side door off Broadway Street, out of the public eye. Wright's Drug Store was on the first floor of the building; in order to reach the college's administrative offices and the lecture hall on the second floor, students had to ascend an enclosed stairwell at the back of the drug store. The dissection laboratory was on the third floor. In light of the neighbors' wariness and suspicion, even animosity, toward the school, the relatively secluded back entrance served them well. The druggist didn't care for the arrangement, but he didn't have much choice: A.C. Remmel owned the building, and he sat on the new college's board of directors.

Two months after the term began, on a crisp Monday morning, the newly appointed demonstrator of anatomy at the school, Dr. Aaron Elliott Van Buskirk, shuffled through a layer of dry maple leaves that had accumulated against that side door and trudged up the dark stairwell in back of the building. Van Buskirk probably hadn't noticed the leaves crunching beneath his feet because he had other things on his mind: he had been summoned to meet with the college's administration. It wasn't likely that the doctors had assembled to discuss the autumnal beauty or to compliment him for his performance during the first two months of the school year. The young doctor's adventure in academic medicine wasn't proceeding as he had envisioned; he was glad he had kept open his little office in town.

During the preceding weeks, the local newspapers had reported that members of the medical college faculty were squabbling among themselves over authority and money, but particularly about their difficulties in obtaining anatomical subjects. Several of the senior doctors pressed their new demonstrator to obtain more student "dissection material." Rumors circulated within the community of Fort Wayne that changes in the administration of the medical college were contemplated. A.E. was in an untenable situation: the school had only opened its doors the year before, and A.E. Van Buskirk was the newest and the youngest faculty member. He reported to the professor of anatomy, Harold A. Clark, who had been his professor of chemistry at Cincinnati's Medical College of Ohio just two years earlier. Undoubtedly, Clark had encouraged his student to accept the position in Fort Wayne after his graduation in 1876. A.E. hoped soon to succeed Clark as professor, for it was clear that the dour chemist didn't have a taste for the business of anatomy—he left every detail to his youthful demonstrator including, and especially, the acquisition of cadavers. Clark rarely made an appearance on the third floor, but A.E. had to prove his mettle before he could receive his mentor's title. To compound his difficulties, the doctors had named A.E. secretary of faculty before the term had even begun, planting upon his naïve, if willing, shoulders the many unpleasant tasks of mediating not only among the doctors but also between the school and an increasingly skeptical community at large.

In its second autumnal term, the school's favor with the citizens of Fort Wayne had faded with the summer leaves. Regardless of any high purpose, the odious dismemberment of corpses over Wright's Drug Store had chilled the spine of the collective community. People crossed the street to avoid the Remmel Building and sometimes complained of fetid aromas that fouled the surrounding neighborhood. To make matters worse, faculty members were at odds with each other over control of the school and over accountability for the paucity of subjects to dissect. Had a recent widow known that during the Monday morning of her husband's funeral, the medical college faculty had convened that day's special meeting specifically to confront their newly appointed demonstrator of anatomy about his deficiencies, she might have been even more wary about the sanctity of her husband's new grave.

A.E. opened the oaken door at the rear of the second floor hall and entered a small conference room. Muted morning sunlight checkered the surface of the round oak table, resulting in a crisp shadow of mullioned windows ominously marking the austere men assembled there. Several of the senior doctors, the very men who had urged A.E. so assiduously to join the faculty of the fledgling school, asked the young doctor to seat himself. Then they began their litany of disputations. His older colleagues complained that there were no cadavers lying upon the tables in the dissection laboratory upstairs.

To make matters worse, several zealous medical students had registered a formal complaint to the school's board of directors about a lack of subject material for the teaching of anatomy.

In 1877, laboratory experience for medical students consisted almost entirely of dissecting human cadavers. Decades behind their colleagues in Europe, North American physicians had barely begun to explore the new fields of microbiology and chemistry, and the quality of medical schools was measured exclusively by the amount of firsthand experience in human anatomical dissection that they could offer their students. The professors reiterated to the young demonstrator that, although he was a member of the faculty, he was, to date, failing in his primary duty that was to procure cadavers and supervise their dissection. There could be no supervision and no teaching when there were no bodies to dissect. The faculty emphasized that the very existence of the college depended on his ability to acquire cadavers. Students who were complaining about their academic deprivation so early in the term could toll the death knell not only for the demonstrator's position, but also for the medical college itself.

The chastised A.E. Van Buskirk promised to do better. When he was dismissed, he plodded down the stairway and headed onto Washington Street toward the town center, contemplating his fate. A.E. had no doubt about his duty. He had been as assiduous in obtaining cadavers as he possibly could have been, but he couldn't very well manufacture a corpse. In a pique of self-indulgence, he wondered if next they would encourage him to emulate the infamous William Burke of Edinburgh who, in 1829, was hanged in connection with several heinous murders and the subsequent sale of the bodies as cadavers for anatomy study. (*See Ch. 6.*)

With his normally rational mind so morbidly obscured, A.E. nearly stumbled when his pace was forcibly slowed to allow passage of what could only be described as a fortuitous procession of mourners. A cortege filed before him, heading toward the Lutheran cemetery on Maumee Road. It didn't take much effort for Dr. Van Buskirk, already attired in his customary black suit, to assume his most somber countenance as he stepped in pace with the crowd. No one seemed to notice that he'd joined the procession or that, as they passed through the iron gate of the graveyard, the anatomist took his place behind the mourners who crowded around the open grave. A.E. watched as the heavily veiled widow dropped a handful of the local black soil onto the coffin of her late husband. The officiating minister seemed to drone for hours, but finally, eulogies completed, the mourners dispersed to their homes. The anatomist hung back a bit, noting in his mind the precise location of the grave, relative to the standing trees, the fence, and the roadside. He immediately returned to the college on Broadway and Washington.

Flushed with newfound anticipation, A.E. directly sought out his inquisitors of that morning to present his good news, but, contradictorily, those same gentlemen who had so severely scolded him just hours before, now advised him to leave that particular body alone. They explained that the deceased had been a beloved citizen whose grave would be guarded carefully. They feared that taking his body would "raise a terrible commotion" in the city.

A.E. did not like their advice. He knew only too well that if he didn't obtain some subjects soon, his career would end before it really had begun. He also thought it duplicitous that some of those same faculty who had threatened him for his inaction now became fastidious about which bodies to take. He decided to ignore their admonitions.

The exact sequence of activities between the time that A.E. left the college for the second time that day and the midnight adventure that he undertook to Emanuel Lutheran Cemetery—with the hired drayman and the medical students—was never precisely established. However, the sequence of events undoubtedly followed the same routine that had been in place since the beginning of the term. Medical students who were assigned to the anatomy laboratory would be notified. A professional "exhumation" would be arranged. It was the same at other medical schools around the country where effective training required fresh cadavers. Because the law provided no good legal means for their acquisition, a sufficient number of bodies could be obtained only one way: by means of a shovel on a dark night and the disreputable skills of a professional body snatcher known as a "resurrectionist." Arrangements needed to be made for delivery of the cadaver.

But on that occasion, apparently because of the short notice, A.E. had to deviate slightly from the usual practice in that there would be no direct exchange between the resurrectionist and his clients at the medical college. Rather, the doctors would be instructed to simply pick up a bagged corpse left inside the graveyard, out of sight from casual passersby. As far as the doctors were to know, the body thief might have had more than one job that night, or he never dallied for a delivery. After all, it was the season of resurrection; his time was valuable.

After notifying the students that he needed three of them to help, Dr. Van Buskirk went to Fletcher and Powers Livery on Barr Street and reserved a wagon and driver for that same evening. He returned before midnight, at which time he helped the drayman hitch the team to the wagon before they set out in the direction of Emanuel Lutheran Cemetery. As they approached the graveyard, A.E. ordered the driver to stop and wait in the darkness of a low ravine. The iron fence of the Lutheran Cemetery loomed just beyond. Alighting from the wagon, A.E. greeted the three medical students. One of them was a giant of fellow, well known in the city as "Big" Sommers. A.E. and the three students crept to the iron fence. Though no one else seemed to be out on the clear cool night, they worked as quickly and as silently as possible. Precisely where the resurrectionist had promised, the doctors found a long sack inside the cemetery, lying on the ground against the wrought iron pickets. It appeared to contain a body. Two of students climbed over the fence and dropped to the ground on the other side. They handed the bulky parcel up and over the barricade to the others who lugged it back to the wagon and heaved it onto the wagon bed. The two who had climbed the fence joined them, and the four men then climbed aboard. A.E. again assumed his seat next to the driver whom he instructed to head back toward town, but that time to go by way of Wayne Street toward the home of one of the professors, where they stopped for Big Sommers to disembark. The remaining two students proceeded with their demonstrator and the draymen to the medical college on the corner of Washington and Broadway. Once they'd stopped there, Van Buskirk and his students unloaded the body, still in its sack, which they lugged through the side door of the building and up the stairs to the college rooms. And the driver returned to his stables.

Despite its seeming spontaneity, the resurrection of Diedrich Buck from the Emanuel Lutheran Cemetery on the night of Monday, November 19, 1877, had transpired without complications.

Like so many undetected body snatches, before and after, it would
never have been discovered were it not for the drayman's chance
remark some months later.

At the time, however, Dr. Van Buskirk arose early in the
morning, feeling rather smug about his actions of the night
before. His colleagues had demanded more subjects and he had
delivered one that was now lying in place on a table in the third
floor laboratory. He completed his morning ablutions as quickly as
possible and headed directly from his home in Monroeville to the
college.

After helping the students begin their work on the new
cadaver, the young anatomist immediately sought Professor
of Surgery William H. Myers, who, by the sheer force of his
personality, had become the *ipso facto* head of the college regardless
of any administrative titles or political events that always swirled
about him. Van Buskirk spoke with Myers in the secretary's office,
coyly inquiring if the surgeon planned to go out to the Lutheran
Cemetery and then, not without some sense of accomplishment,
he told the older man that he didn't wish the professor to dig into
an empty grave. He revealed that he had been there himself to take
the body the night before.

Professor Myers had undoubtedly been among those who
had reprimanded the demonstrator for the paucity of anatomical
subjects but, perhaps, had also cautioned him against taking the
particular body of Diedrich Buck. However, in the morning light,
in the absence of any evident discovery of the snatch, Myers could
do little but nod encouragement to his young demonstrator. Van
Buskirk was surely disappointed if he expected some gratuitous
accolade for his nocturnal acquisition, for the surgeon was as short
with his compliments as he was generous with his complaints.

Myers was one of the most contentious members of the faculty,
but he was also one of the most powerful and influential. The
medical students respected none of the faculty more than their
professor of surgery. A junior faculty member such as Dr. Van

Buskirk needed Myers's support to maintain his position within the school. To make matters more difficult, though Myers had hired A.E. from Monroeville, they had immediately crossed swords when Van Buskirk, in his capacity as secretary of the faculty, had been called upon to challenge the gruff surgeon a few weeks earlier and had found himself caught between the polarized factions of the college with Myers leading the charge against the antagonists. The news of the fresh cadaver seemed to mollify the professor because it tempered, for the time being, the students' protestations; they put their grumblings aside as they began a fresh dissection in earnest.

Myers later reported that he and Van Buskirk went to the anatomy laboratory together where they found some students working on what was by then a partially dissected cadaver. Myers observed that the body was distinctive because of the severe deformation of the second toe on the left foot. He demanded a hammer and bone chisel from one of the students and promptly amputated the distorted toe with a swift single blow to its base. He then turned to Dr. Van Buskirk, who'd been startled by the unceremonious severance of his cadaver's appendage, and reiterated the school's policy of obliterating all identifying characteristics from the cadavers as soon as they arrived on the table. Ignoring the implicit reprimand, the young demonstrator nodded his agreement, then drew the surgeon's attention to the subject's right inguinal hernia. They decided that the hernia was a common enough malady that it didn't require special attention.

The local newspapers regularly reported the existence of bodies upon the tables in the college as well as suspected robberies of the local graveyards. Although the obvious association was lost on no one, the school, thus far, had successfully maintained that all of their cadavers had been shipped to Fort Wayne from out of town. Nonetheless, Myers was well aware that the laboratory could be inspected at any time, and he required extreme caution in all instances.

But that afternoon when Myers lopped off the toe, after which the dissection continued to progress without difficulty, A.E. left with Myers to attend his own clinics, satisfied that he had held at bay the admonitions of his colleagues. His mind then cleared, the young anatomist stopped on Calhoun Street at a newsstand where one of the columns in the afternoon paper caught his eye. It proclaimed that a prominent local gardener, Charles Wright, lay near death in his home along the banks of the White River, north of the city.

CHAPTER 6

The Body Snatchers

THE PRACTICE OF DISSECTING human cadavers, whether unclaimed bodies or the remains of fallen warriors, nobility, or even holy men, dates to the earliest antiquity, but the crime of body snatching to obtain subjects for anatomic dissection was a peculiarly Anglo-Saxon institution. Neither Protestant nor Catholic dogma specifically prohibited anatomic dissection, but many believed that a body torn asunder would drift forever in purgatory, denied passage through the holy gates. Nearly a century earlier than in Great Britain, the practice of human dissection became established on the European continent where bodies were provided to anatomists and artists. These were often granted by royal proclamation as a convenient method for discouraging crime, disposing of unclaimed bodies, and encouraging the advancement of science and art, all at the same time.

British teaching of anatomy began in the late fourteenth century, primarily among barber surgeons who wanted to advance their skills within their trade. By an act of parliament during the reign of Henry VIII, the English crown provided bodies of executed felons, at first four per year, a number that later increased to six. The ignobility of dissection could be added to the sentence of execution as a further punishment that, in the minds of the condemned and their survivors, reached beyond the grave. These dissections of executed criminals, by law, took place publicly, in so-called "public anatomies," in the hall of the Company of Barber Surgeons. Attendance was open to anyone, but it was required for the members of the barber guild. At each public session, three bodies were dissected: one for muscles, one for bones, and one for the internal organs. Any other dissection was forbidden. Interested academics who chafed under the ban against their own firsthand observation, often performed illicit dissections in their own private chambers.

In eighteenth-century England, the Corporation of Surgeons required demonstration of anatomic proficiency by the satisfactory completion of two courses of dissection to qualify as a surgeon, though no legal means existed to acquire the requisite cadavers. The aspiring surgeons had no recourse except to troll the local graveyards under the cover of darkness. Dissection of cadavers had become such a vital foundation block of medical education that students, preceptors, and professors of anatomy risked their licenses, their reputations, and even their lives to obtain their subjects. The teachers of anatomy competed among one another to attract students by guaranteeing the availability of well-preserved and interesting bodies for dissection. As the demand expanded, the occasional nocturnal sojourn of a medical student to the local graveyard became insufficient to meet the need. Even the most august of professors were compelled to contract with professional body thieves to assure a steady supply of subjects.

Such "resurrectionists" organized to meet the needs. By 1820, local authorities estimated that half a dozen people in London devoted their full vocational time to providing cadavers for anatomists, but gangs of part-time body thieves competed with the "professionals." The resurrectionists normally had an arrangement with the night supervisor of the graveyard who would leave the gate open and assure that the workers were not disturbed. When found out, the men usually lost their job at the cemetery only to join the ranks of the body snatchers themselves.

Many of the medical schools established their own museums of interesting specimens, the most famous of which was founded by John Hunter and is, in part, preserved today at the Royal College of Surgeons in London. John and his brother William were avid anatomists and collectors of specimens, human and otherwise. John Hunter was a pioneer of modern surgery, but is equally remembered for his eccentricity and for the museum of anatomic specimens that he maintained at his home in Earl's Court. Hunter once went so far as to arrange for a dying 7' 7" Irish pituitary giant named Charles Byrne to be stalked, day and night, so that his body could be harvested for the Hunterian Museum. Byrne, horrified by the prospect, arranged that his corpse would be guarded and buried in a lead coffin at sea. When he died, the undertaker made all the arrangements, but Hunter's men bribed the pallbearers when they stopped at a roadhouse. As the coffin, weighted with rocks, dropped into the sea, its former occupant rode in Hunter's own carriage to Earl's Court. Despite vociferous contemporary ethical controversy, Byrne's huge skeleton still hung in the Hunterian Museum of the Royal College of Surgeons in London until the museum closed for renovations in 2017.

The leading anatomists such as Joshua Brookes and Sir Astley Cooper contracted with specific resurrection agents to assure a regular supply of material. They were forced to pay an advance retainer for the thieves' availability during the laboratory season, a per-body fee ranging from 4 to as much as 16 guineas, and a delivery fee. In addition, the anatomist often paid bail for the apprehended resurrectionist, trial costs, and even family support during jail time. Eventually, the surgeons organized a College of Anatomy in an unsuccessful attempt to establish affordable resurrection prices. The college petitioned both the parliament and the public about the absurdity of obliging the teachers to resort to criminal activity to obtain subject materials. They emphasized the necessity of learning anatomy to become a physician; Sir Astley Cooper even made his famous comparison of a surgeon who had not done dissection to a watchmaker who had never examined the workings of a watch. Several proposals came forth, including one that would have required debtors, prostitutes, and the poor to become candidates for dissection after death. Those singled out were terrified in contemplation of dismemberment of their corporal remains. Anyone unfortunate enough to be poor could be, according to some religious beliefs, eternally stamped with the stigma of crime and ultimately barred from the gates of heaven.

By the late 1820s, the demand for cadavers ran so high that even the professional body thieves were having trouble filling their orders. They began to look beyond the dead, to the street urchins roaming the back alleys. The most famous case of Burke and Hare in Scotland seared its imprint on the English lexicon when "to burke" came to mean, "to murder for gain."

In 1827, William Burke and William Hare began as dealers in bodies for the dissection rooms in Edinburgh. One of their subjects had, in life, owed Hare 4£. For Burke and Hare, waiting for their debtor's natural demise became an unacceptable encumbrance when they knew they could collect 7£ for his body from any of the various anatomy laboratories—so, they smothered him in his sleep. For the next year, Burke and Hare embarked upon a series of undetected murders among the street people of Edinburgh. They delivered these fresh cadavers to the anatomists, principally Alexander Munro, the first chair of anatomy at the University of Edinburgh, and Robert Knox, a promising young anatomist who ran his own dissecting rooms nearby.

Burke and Hare's downfall came with the report of a stinking body in their rooms, which was, in fact, awaiting delivery. When the police arrived, the body was gone but was subsequently discovered, still in its sealed box, in the rooms of the anatomist, Robert Knox. Burke and Hare were arrested. Hare turned state's evidence; Burke was convicted and hanged with the stipulation that his body was to undergo public dissection.

A throng turned out for both the hanging and the dissection. Hare had been released for testifying against Burke, but he quickly escaped Scotland with his life. Eventually, he was caught in England by a vigilante mob and thrown into a vat of lye. He survived, only to live another forty years as a blind beggar in London. Both the court and a professional investigating committee had exonerated the anatomist, Robert Knox, but Knox became the public scapegoat. He was passed over as the chair of anatomy and was forced to leave Edinburgh. Knox lived the remainder of his life in relative obscurity. In fact, Knox had received the body quite by accident. Hare had brought the corpse to the university for delivery to Professor Munro, but he was intercepted by one of Knox's well-meaning students.

After a similar case of "burking"—which usually involved smothering—the public demanded legislative reform. The Anatomy Act, passed in 1832, obviated the nefarious market for bodies by stating that every body that went unclaimed after forty-eight hours would be provided to a hospital or private anatomy school. The remains were to be buried at the recipient school's expense.

Decades earlier, in 1750, Thomas Cadwalader (1708–1779) of Philadelphia had offered the first course of dissection in North America. In that same year, in New York City, Drs. John Bard and Peter Middleton dissected the body of an executed criminal "for the instruction of the young men then engaged in the study of medicine." William Shippen and fellow Philadelphian John Morgan founded the first American medical college as the College of Philadelphia where Shippen became the first professor of anatomy in 1765. The opening of his anatomic theatre incited such alarm among Philadelphians that his sessions were interrupted several times by public riots, during one of which the professor had to escape through a back alley.

As had transpired in England until the Anatomy Act of 1832, the only legal source of bodies for dissection in post-revolutionary America had come from executions. Again, these failed to meet the needs of the medical colleges and stamped the endeavor of anatomic dissection with the disgrace of a condemned criminal. The public so strongly associated the teaching of medicine with the robbing of graves that they invariably enacted provisions to prohibit the practice whenever they chartered a new a college of medicine. The stigma lasted well into the waning days of the resurrectionists when, a century later, Ambrose Bierce defined a grave as "a place in which the dead are laid to await the coming of the medical student."[18]

But a medical college could not exist without an adequate supply of cadavers. The majority of subjects that were dissected in medical colleges of North America had been obtained illegally from financial arrangements between the teachers of anatomy and professional "resurrectionists." Of the 400 bodies dissected by the medical colleges in Vermont between 1820 and 1840, only 40 came from legal sources. Most "resurrections" went undetected, or perhaps unnoticed by people who intentionally looked the other way.

Although the responsibility for procuring bodies rested upon the professor or demonstrator of anatomy, the actual work fell to the lay professionals who had acquired the same skill and daring of their British resurrectionist predecessors.

The robbing of graves in early America had become a highly profitable and organized business among professionals who followed the techniques for disinterment and disposition of the body similar to those established in Great Britain in previous decades. These methods were designed to prevent identification of the perpetrators and to conceal that the grave robbery had taken place. Because of the need for relatively fresh material, bodies were usually taken during the first night after the burial; the resurrectionists tended to choose cemeteries that were relatively isolated from homes and

---

18 Ambrose Bierce, *The Devil's Dictionary*, 1911 edition (Cornell University Library, 2009).

buildings. They preferred to invade the "potter's field," that portion of cemeteries reserved for burials at public expense, because those areas tended to be more remote and less likely to be visited.[19] As the demand for fresh cadavers intensified, no cemetery was spared. It was a rare burial, regardless of the social standing of the bereaved, that a resurrection was not at least contemplated.

The first recorded body snatching in Ohio occurred at Zanesville in 1811 when an open grave was discovered and wheelbarrow tracks led from there to a hotel basement where three apprenticed medical students lived. The townspeople broke into the hotel's cellar and found the body hidden behind some logs. Despite the wishes of the mob, no arrest could be made because a dead body did not constitute property. Following the precedents of English law, only the removal of the shroud or any other property could be construed to be felonious. For that reason, body snatchers were scrupulous about leaving all property undisturbed.

Later, in 1845, the stench arising from a shipping box addressed to a doctor in Cleveland caused it to be opened; it revealed the bodies of a woman and a child, taken from graves in Austinburg, Ohio. The local Reverend S.W. Streeter of the Congregational Church condemned grave robbing in the strongest of terms from his pulpit, but, at the same time, he called for the passage of legislation that would provide dissection material to medical schools to assure adequate training of doctors. Such legislation would have to wait nearly another forty years to be passed in Ohio.[20]

There can be no question that A.E. Van Buskirk was exposed to grave robbing while a student in Ohio, both in Wooster and in

---

19 The term, "potter's field" derives from Judas Iscariot being repentant when he returned to the priests the 30 pieces of silver he had received for his betrayal of Jesus. The priests felt the tainted money could not be returned to the treasury and, instead, decreed that it would be used to buy a plot of land in Jerusalem for the burial of strangers. The land chosen had been the site of an abandoned pottery.

20 Linden F. Edwards, *Body Snatching in 19th Century Ohio*, prepared by the staff of the Library of Fort Wayne and Allen County, 1955. (The author believes that this was originally from *The Ohio State Archaeological and Historical Quarterly*, 1950.)

Cincinnati. The topic was on the mind of everyone who lived near medical colleges. Newspapers decried the practice in their pages; preachers, from their pulpits. In Cincinnati, body snatchings were a nearly daily occurrence and often went undetected.

The numerous medical colleges were well supplied with cadavers. In October 1875, the bodies of a man and a woman were taken from the German Protestant Cemetery in Cincinnati and delivered to the Medical College of Ohio while Van Buskirk was a student there. Police with search warrants entered the school, broke down the locked doors of the dissecting laboratory, and nearly instituted a riot among the medical students, requiring reinforcements to quell the uprising.

CHAPTER 7

The Death of Charles Wright

I
N 1872, AFTER A LONG PASSAGE four years earlier from England to New York City, Charles Wright, his wife, Mary, and their three children moved to Fort Wayne. By the time the Wrights arrived, many of the hardy settlers from Pennsylvania and Ohio, especially those of German descent, had already become Fort Wayne's leading citizens. They'd established successful businesses and founded opera, music, and theatre. And then they wanted English gardens to grace their grand homes and fine hotels.

Charles Wright, an English gardener, was the man to provide them. By 1877, he'd established a prosperous nursery business, and he had even applied for naturalization to become a full citizen in his adopted land.

Soon after arriving in Fort Wayne, Wright purchased riverfront property north of town, which was ideally suited for his gardening business. The waterways and rich black river bottom soil provided ready access to the supplies he needed but would not prove beneficial in other ways. As was common among the pioneers who situated their settlements along the western riverbanks, the Wrights had inadvertently chosen disease-ridden, lowland swamps for their homesteads. Because communities like Fort Wayne were situated in those swamps, the area was ravaged by periodic epidemics. Waves of cholera, diarrhea (flux), and fevers of every sort cut a scythe swath from house to house, taking one child, one family, and moving on to the next.

In response, at the first sign of contagion, many of the residents evacuated the city as if from an invading army. To escape the pestilence, they would run to their cottages or farmhouses in the surrounding countryside, which were on higher ground, away from the swamps, the bugs, and the filth of the city. Just about everyone who was able left town, often staying with relative farmers or simply begging for a few days lodging in the barn of a kind stranger until the sickness passed.

During the well-documented cholera epidemic of 1849, 1,600 of the 2,000 residents of Aurora, Indiana, fled for the healthier countryside. There was little doubt in the minds of most ordinary people about the source of these contagions. The overriding belief held that the noxious miasma that wafted in the air over swamps, lowland water, and urban gutters produced toxic gases that poisoned the atmosphere and anyone who breathed it. Even physicians clung to the miasmatic theory of illness, whereby malaria, yellow fever, cholera, and a host of others were attributed to poisons in the air wafting over the decaying organic material in swamps and areas of organic filth. The germ theory of disease was slow to reach the western frontier; it was still just a crazy idea in the minds of most who had heard of it. But the idea that the very air they breathed carried the diseases compelled the citizenry of the Midwest to keep their houses tightly shut from the noxious gases festering outside. One pioneer woman's pathetic letter questioned how her child could have died when they had been so careful to keep the windows and doors tightly shut.

Unknowingly, the miasmatics almost had it right—except that miasma had nothing to do with it. Each epidemic had its own hidden vector: the urban filth of the open sewers and latrines contaminated the drinking water with cholera; the crowded conditions concentrated the airborne micro-droplets of tubercle bacilli; the stagnant water in the swamps, ponds, and rain barrels attracted the mosquitoes that carried malaria and yellow fever. In fact, the riversides were so dense with mosquitoes that the early settlers told stories about evening clouds of bugs so thick that when one held an arm out and quickly withdrew it, a visible cavity would be left in the insect-laden atmosphere. Malarial fever had become a natural part of the western settler's life. One pioneer wrote home that the population, in spite of the hard life, was remarkably healthy, except, "of course, for fever."

Wright's land lay in perhaps the worst of all locations, between the river and a great stagnant pond. Little did Charles understand that he had chosen a virtual paradise for pestilent nesting mosquitoes. Like many newcomers with no natural immunity, he'd contracted malaria (intermittent fever or *ague* as it was commonly known), almost as soon as he'd arrived. He and Mary really had not thought much about it; most of the people they knew had had a touch of fever now and then. Their family physician, Dr. Benjamin Woodworth, told them they must get away from the pestilential lowland gases, but Charles and Mary were in no position to move. They had barely established their family in Fort Wayne, and they'd just come through the depression of 1873. To let the gardens go bad would have devastated their business.

Dr. Benjamin Woodworth, one of Fort Wayne's first and most admired physicians, was among the most accessible of doctors to the new ideas in medicine; he was the strongest advocate for change when it seemed indicated. He also was among the first and most outspoken physician against the poisonous "heroic" regimens of the antebellum era when gargantuan doses of mercury or arsenic were as likely to maim or kill as they were to save. But for all his grace and sophistication, Benjamin Woodworth clung to the idea of miasma borne disease.

By the time of Charles Wright's sickness in 1877, the concept of bacteria-induced illness was well established among the medical leaders in Britain and continental Europe, but the majority of American doctors remained aggressively skeptical, scoffing at the idea of microscopic organisms causing disease. Only the year before, in September 1876, during the Philadelphia Centennial Exhibition, Joseph Lister, the surgeon to Queen Victoria, whose methods of antiseptic surgery had been widely embraced across the Atlantic, addressed the leading American surgeons at the University of Pennsylvania. He had been invited by one of nation's most prominent surgeons, Samuel Gross, to present his antiseptic surgical methods before the International Medical Congress. Sadly, despite an erudite and lengthy discussion of the germ theory for the putrefaction of wounds, Lister's word fell on deaf ears and elicited mainly diatribes against his ideas and even imputations of his character.[21] Most practicing nineteenth-century physicians viewed the germ theory of disease as a kind of arcane philosophy that was more interesting to contemplate than to actually have any practical application to their sick and dying patients.

In one of his lucid moments, Charles ruminated over Doc Woodworth's claim that the very ground and the air above it festered with the filth of fever. On top of ague, Charles complained of swellings on his neck and head. At first, they really didn't hurt, but they gave him a lumpy, grotesque, appearance. With the summer past, the cooler weather seemed to quiet Charles's fever, but not the scrofula festering in his neck and scalp. By fall, the tumors had spread all over his head; their effluvium seeped into his bedclothes. Woodworth had wanted to cut out the biggest tumor on his neck, but Charles had been afraid. Even with the new chloroform sleeping gas to ease the pain, many died from septic infection after surgery. Some of the evil masses began painfully to break through the skin, oozing their repulsive purulence. Dr. Woodworth told the Wrights that those were the lesions of scrofula, tuberculosis of lymph glands in the neck. After decades of medical practice in

---

21 Physicians in New York, Boston, and Chicago were far more accepting, but it would not be until the end of the century before Lister's methods would be widely adopted in the United States. Lindsey Fitzharris, *The Butchering Art: Joseph Lister's Quest to Transform the Grisly World of Victorian Medicine* (New York, NY: Scientific American / Farrar, Straus and Giroux, 2017), 219–221.

the region, the doctor found Charles's condition morbidly serious, but not particularly unusual or mysterious. He saw patients like Charles every day. As he was to testify later, it had never occurred to him to request a consultation for such an ordinary condition.

Dr. Woodworth specifically and publicly insisted upon his diagnosis of Charles Wright as chronic malaria complicated in the final year of life by scrofula. The scrofulous lymph gland was as easily recognizable by Benjamin Woodworth in the nineteenth century by its firm rubbery texture and lack of tenderness as it was by his successors in the twenty-first century. This finding would contrast with the abscesses that were also observed and lanced by Dr. Woodworth, but secondary infection with other bacteria could easily lead to the kind of abscesses that he had described. The elementary distinction between the fluctuant abscess and the firm rubbery granuloma of scrofula left no room for confusion in Dr. Woodworth's mind about Wright's diagnosis. He did speculate that one of the abscesses may have invaded the carotid artery, the main blood supply to the brain, and caused a stroke. (Today, such a catastrophe would be recognized as a "septic" or infectious embolus, a chunk of pustulate debris adrift in the arterial blood stream to the brain.) In his description of Wright's final illness in the Fort Wayne newspaper, Woodworth makes no specific mention of ever having considered Charles's malaria as contributory to his death. Malaria is associated with obstructions of the blood flow to vital areas and seems, in retrospect, as likely as a scrofulous invasion of the carotid artery as suggested by Dr. Woodworth. When called upon to defend his treatment of Charles Wright in the *Fort Wayne Daily News* of November 28, Woodworth expressed no reservation about his diagnosis of Charles's illness; it did not occur to him to order an autopsy. Perhaps, in reality, he knew that an "autopsy" had already been planned.

Regardless of the exact chain of pathologic, inexorable events within his body, for the last three weeks of his life, Charles Wright waxed in and out of restless consciousness, punctuated by convulsive seizures. Beyond lancing the abscesses, Dr. Woodworth could offer nothing much except to rest his patient, keeping him as comfortable as possible, and allowing Mother Nature to follow her inevitable course.

By 1877, American medical practice was in the peculiar situation of having discarded the horrific bleeding, purging, and blistering of the antebellum era, but having developed few practical remedies to take their place. For some, the idea of specifically treating an illness was considered a sacrilege, equivalent to striking the hand of God. Several more decades of scientific investigation would be needed before organ- or agent-specific treatments would be available and acceptable to the majority of doctors and their patients.

Roberts Bartholow, professor of *materia medica* at the prestigious Medical College of Ohio in Cincinnati, had taught many of the Fort Wayne physicians and had written the definitive textbook, *A Practical Treatise on Materia Medica and Therapeutics*, about disease therapeutics. Bartholow's 1884 edition called for the extract from the root of the Peruvian cinchona bark, quinine, as the most specific and important treatment for malaria. It was one of the few specific drugs available for any disease and remained the primary preventative and therapeutic agent against malaria until World War II. For scrofula, Bartholow prescribed cod-liver oil and inunction of oil, with phosphates to improve nutrition with iron with chalybeate waters. "Iodides of iron and manganese, especially stillingia, sanguinaria, and sarsaparilla promote activity of the vegetative functions."[22] Other than the quinine for his malaria, these agents served mainly as irritants to the bowel or skin and did little from our contemporary viewpoint except exacerbate the patient's misery and perhaps hasten his demise.

Dr. Woodworth advised Mary Wright to prepare for the worst. There wasn't much else to be done except to keep him clean and

---

22 Roberts Bartholow, *A Practical Treatise on Materia Medica and Therapeutics*, 5th ed. (New York, NY: D. Appleton and Company, 1884).

comfortable. It would not be long. On Monday, November 19, 1877, even as the demonstrator of anatomy was on his way to the Lutheran cemetery on Maumee Road, Charles Wright closed his eyes, perhaps for the last time, his face in relative repose. His daughter Charlotte went to the oak wardrobe and pulled out his best suit that they'd bought from Pixley's store on Berry Street. She hung it on the clothes tree in the upstairs hall to take down to old Mr. Peltier. Wright lapsed into unconsciousness for the last time on November 21. By Thursday morning, November 22, Charles Wright, English gardener of Fort Wayne, Indiana, had died. All of the funeral arrangements, by then, had been made.

CHAPTER 8

The Interment

J.C. PELTIER HAD HEARD that Charles Wright had been clinging to life far beyond anyone's expectations, wasting, and oozing into his bed down by the river. The Peltier family was one of the oldest in Fort Wayne. J.C.'s father, Louis Peltier, had been born in the old stockade and established his undertaking business in 1845.

Louis Peltier and Son, Undertakers, at 17 W. Wayne Street, were the best undertakers in town and would take care of everything for the family of Charles Wright. Louis Peltier and Son knew a good funeral. The senior Peltier had given an interview to the *Fort Wayne Weekly Sentinel* a few years earlier, in which he had affirmed that funerals in Fort Wayne were "as well conducted as in any city in the country."[23] As had been true since establishment of the elaborate funereal customs in pharaonic Egypt, funerals in nineteenth-century Fort Wayne varied widely in preparation, elaboration, and cost, depending upon the wealth and status of the deceased and the circumstances of his or her death. Peltier priced a "county funeral" at $10, including a pine box, a plain hearse, and no carriages. Carriages were reserved for "inmates of the hospital and asylum, victims of accidents, and the many poor and worthy people." The most popular funeral choice ran between $20 and $30

---

23 *Fort Wayne Weekly Sentinel*, June 9, 1875.

and was somewhat more elaborate with a walnut coffin, a hearse, and a carriage.

Peltier noted that, "A nice coffin and hearse with two or three carriages" ran $50 to $60. Much more expensive variations were also available and, for everyone, cemetery plots were additional. To complicate matters, public fear of body snatching had spawned a whole new industry of theft-proof coffins, from completely iron caskets to those with explosive-charged lids designed to maim or kill the interlopers.[24] In Charles Wright's case, Mr. Peltier felt the wooden coffin would be more than adequate because he believed that Charles's emaciation would obviate much interest in his body for student dissection.

Peltier arranged to pick up Charles's body from the home, deliver it directly to the Trinity Episcopal Church on Berry Street, and lead the cortege to the cemetery. He would also provide Mary with a mourning carriage that would have black plumes projecting from each corner of the top. He advised that they purchase her a mourning dress; she would wear black for a while, so the investment was probably worthwhile.

American mourning customs followed the English who were deeply influenced by Queen Victoria's profound and prolonged mourning of her beloved Prince Albert. The standards were somewhat less stringent in America, but a widow often was expected to wear full mourning dress for a year and a day; this meant a dull, black, unadorned dress and a "weeping" veil. Some exceptions could be made for working women such as Mary, but the period of full mourning would not have been less than six months.

Mr. Peltier advised that, considering the condition of Charles's body, they should hold the funeral as soon as possible after his death and forego the customary viewing in their home. The undertaker explained that he would send the carriage to the house to gather the

---

24 Fiona Hutton, *The Study of Anatomy in Britain, 1700–1900* (London and New York: Routledge, 2015).

family about an hour before the church service was to begin, and that he also would make arrangements with the cemetery. Charles would be buried at Lindenwood, the lovely grounds of a 152-acre spread along the old Wabash and Erie Canal on the western edge of town. In 1864, a new road and bridge had been built over the canal to provide better access into the cemetery.

Shaded by massive virginal hardwoods, Lindenwood was originally acquired from the Potawatomi Indians in 1826. George Ewing, one of Fort Wayne's founding entrepreneurs, eventually bought the land and sold it to a consortium of Fort Wayne's wealthier citizens to found Lindenwood Cemetery in 1859. With several others, Fort Wayne's most prominent citizen, Hugh McCulloch, had expressed concern about the paucity of decent burial places in their burgeoning city.

Throughout mid-nineteenth-century America, concerned citizens complained about the unpleasantness, overcrowding, and impropriety of urban graveyards. Politicians urged the passage of ordinances that would require cemeteries to be built on the periphery of the towns. The new Lindenwood board of directors hired a young English landscape architect, John Doswell, to serve as superintendent of the cemetery and to build a beautiful and tranquil place for all who visited, both those above and beneath its wooded grounds. The first burial took place on July 6, 1860. Single cemetery plots sold for $5; the burial of an adult, $4; a child, $2. The board of directors continued to run the cemetery as a private concern until July 1877, when it was transferred to the City of Fort Wayne, a few months before the fall opening of the second medical college fall term.

The papers announced that Charles Wright's funeral was to be held at three o'clock on that November Thursday. Peltier's men already had scrubbed down the hearse, its black enamel glistening even in the gloom of the carriage house. By half past one, the team was hitched, neighing nervously. The attendants pulled on their mourning coats. Coachmen climbed onto the seat as the footmen fell in line alongside, top hats glistening in the mist. The driver set the team on its way, pulling out onto Wayne Street, then to Calhoun, and proceeded six blocks west to the church. Around two o'clock in the afternoon, Peltier's black hearse stopped in the back of Trinity Episcopal Church, a few blocks east of Broadway. By two thirty, Peltier's carriage discharged Mary Wright and the family in front of the church.

The Wright's friends and relatives had known that Charles was dying, so the funeral notice of that morning had been no surprise, but it had held a special interest for a small group of people who were not mourners. Two days earlier, the notice of Wright's terminal sickness on page one of the *Daily News* had already caught the eyes of the medical students on Broadway.

The afternoon was blustery; the gray sky threatened to become drizzly. The family entered the building while the hearse stood in front, waiting for the service to finish. Peltier arranged the cortege to face west. The plan was that they would turn right on Broadway one block and left onto Main before heading to Lindenwood. Peltier's newspaper advertisements pictured the elegant wagon in nearly every edition, but standing right there on the street for an hour or so with the gleaming bier and carriages wouldn't hurt business. (*See Fig. 5.*)

Across the street from the church, a young boy stopped to stare before his mother whisked him inside their frame house. At three thirty, the church doors cracked open; the coachmen sat up smartly. The pallbearers brought the new casket down the steps, carrying their load by wrought iron handles that hung from the iron band around the perimeter of the walnut box. The coffin slid in through the back, brushing the velvet curtains as it passed; the attendants raised the gate to lock it in place. Mary and the family climbed into Peltier's carriage that followed behind. Other mourners fell in line to the rear of the family.

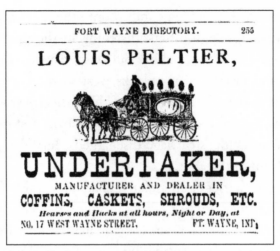

Figure 5. Louis Peltier, Undertaker. Advertisement, Fort Wayne City Directory, *1876–1877.*

Two of the students from the nearby medical college had been lurking about the Trinity Episcopal Church. As the procession trailed past the medical school toward Lindenwood Cemetery, they stepped in line toward the back; they followed the cortege closely enough to be taken for mourners, of which there were many.

The horses maintained a steady clip down Main, over St. Mary's Bridge, and onto the new cemetery road. The carriage rolled over a second bridge that spanned the old canal, and then passed the gate into Lindenwood. Mary no doubt found it sad that so lovely a place was a garden of death. She and Charles had strolled its pathways past the lake and the handsome stone arbors and benches that John Doswell strategically had strewn about and gave an appearance of natural outcroppings of the land. Now Charles was gone; she hoped Doswell would protect his grave.

The procession proceeded beside the newly installed wrought iron fence to the south end of Lindenwood. The road curved between the base of a gentle hill and one of Doswell's creeks on the left. To the right, the roof of a cobblestone gazebo peeked over the crest of the wooded slope. The cortege halted. The guests disembarked for the short walk up the hillside to the grave. Superintendent Doswell was already standing by, looking solemn, reassuringly in charge. Even Isaac D.G. Nelson, president of the Lindenwood board, had attended to pay his respects. The six bearers moved to the rear of the hearse, disengaged the wooden coffin from its wagon crypt, and struggled up the hill toward the grave, which had already been neatly dug by the old sexton. Mary didn't like the sexton's face, which seemed distorted into a sort of permanent sneer. She supposed it was the nature of his business, the years of wincing from the smell of death. Doswell had said he was a gentle, if simple, soul.

By then, the crowd assembled around the sepulcher in what had become the twilight of late November. The two young men from the medical college arrived in time to watch the pallbearers lug the heavy coffin up the hillside. They ascertained it to be constructed of wood, with iron handles that the pallbearers would use to lower it in place. The body, said to be withered to skin, bones, and pustules, probably would not be of much interest, but the professors were putting a lot of pressure on Dr. Van Buskirk to get "subjects." The two students moved to the periphery of the bleak assembly and stood among the tall trees up the hillside from the grave. From there they could see the necessary details but could also duck unobtrusively under the large stone gazebo if they were spotted.

The vicar gave a grand eulogy that Mary Wright didn't really hear. When it was over, the family lingered to drop handfuls of the wet earth on the coffin; then the sexton quickly filled up the void. Doswell murmured sympathies and reiterated his reassurances about the grave. He remained a few moments to oversee the sexton place his mark in the lower right corner on the carefully raked earth, as if it were an amulet that would protect the grave. As Mary and the family turned to go, Doswell reinforced his orders to the sexton for his strictest precautions during the night. By then, they knew that it was usually the first night that a resurrectionist came—while the body was still in prime condition for dissection. But the superintendent had reassured the family that he had taken care of everything. And even Mr. Nelson was there, representing the cemetery board.

After the crowd dispersed, the widow stood with her children a few minutes before taking her final leave. The two men behind the gazebo had watched as Doswell's sexton stamped his mark in the lower right corner; then they moved up, over the crest of the hill. They made a show of visiting another grave and, when the crowd cleared off, they departed by way of Wright's grave for a closer inspection of the mark.

If Charles Wright bore any responsibility for his posthumous fate, it lay in the time he'd picked for his demise, for this was autumn, the season of resurrection. Along with the recommencement of fall classes in the Medical College of Fort Wayne had come the resumption of that sordid, if common, variety of academic supply provided by the local resurrectionist, who had, in fact, already been busy at work earlier in the week.

The druggist, William Wright (no relation to Charles), had also read the front page notice about Charles's terminal illness, and old Dr. Woodworth had confirmed the impending death when he stopped by to drop off some prescriptions. As Wright had done three days earlier in regard to another body, he made his way up the steps in the back of his store to fulfill his arrangement with the school. After all, medical students often first heard of an impending death from a pharmacist. But Wright needn't have bothered; the students already were making preparations.

An impending death invoked a now familiar ritual at the medical college: confirm the time of the funeral, identify the graveyard, contact the "resurrectionist," order the wagon, and prepare for a long night's work. The timing couldn't have been better: the gloomy day foretold a nocturnal fog that would mask the moonlight.

The morning before Wright's funeral, the two students who planned to attend the funeral arranged to meet the resurrectionist at one o'clock the following morning at the southeastern gate of the cemetery, where the road branched along a stream. His package would be waiting for them. The young men had already confirmed with their new demonstrator, Dr. Van Buskirk, that he could expect it.

On their way back into town from the interment that afternoon, the students stopped at the resurrectionist's hovel to advise him of the grave's exact location and other logistics. He confirmed that he would meet them with the corpse at one o'clock, and that they should signal, as usual, with a long whistle. But before the students reached the medical college, they had one more errand: to arrange transportation.

A short walk from Broadway, Fletcher and Powers Livery on Barr Street rented carriages, horses, and wagons, with or without drivers by the hour, the day, or the week. They made regular trips to and from the railroad depot to deliver passengers to the many hotels and boarding houses that had sprouted all over town. Because the students were becoming regular customers, they spoke directly with Mr. Woodward, the manager. They said they would need a wagon and driver for around 11:30 p.m. Woodward summoned his hack driver, Charles Feltz, from the stable. Feltz agreed to meet them with a harnessed rig at the stable gate.

The two men then returned to Washington and Broadway to tell their colleagues at the school that the livery wagon would arrive around one-thirty or two o'clock in the morning; they said they would knock on the side door downstairs when they arrived.

Arrangements completed, the students sat down to wait while some of the others cleared off one of the tables and fired up the old furnace. Later, they ambled up to Anderson's Saloon to take some fortification for the evening. Druggist Wright had closed up at six; all was dark, inside and out. They had made all their contacts; there was nothing left to do but be patient.

Around 11:00 p.m., the two students and a third who might be needed to help transport the load, met their demonstrator of anatomy in front of Wright's Drug Store. Van Buskirk had a couple of smelly old blankets tucked under one arm. Together, the men made their way, on foot, down Washington Street to Calhoun, and then turned on Wayne, right to Fletcher and Powers Livery. The driver, Charles Feltz, seemed unhappy about being involved with hauling bodies, but it was part of his job, and he no doubt needed his pay. He waited at the gate; he was already seated on his wagon at eleven thirty as ordered. Not much was said. The demonstrator, who Feltz called "Doc" heaved the blankets into the back of the wagon and climbed onto the seat beside Feltz. One student sat beside the doctor; the two other students jumped in the back, keeping their distance from the foul covers. A sick amber aura rimmed the gaslights on the street corners; the horse snorted with presentiment.

Meanwhile, the last horsecar made its way up the tracks on Calhoun Street. Most of the street traffic had long since retired for the night. The damp chill in the air might have discouraged other, less ardent students; it penetrated the bones of the living and the dead and blurred the distinction. But it wasn't the first time for such nocturnal adventure, although it always left a queasy feeling in their stomachs. There had to be a better way to learn the structures.

The doctor gave the word, and they headed out onto the street. The wagon soon passed beyond the muted streetlights to the darkened west side of town along Main. No one spoke. Feltz knew the way; so did the horse. Where they crossed Broadway, they could see, about one block south of the school, Anderson's Hotel, where Madame Mariotte rented rooms by the hour. A few revelers hung around in front of Goodwin's Dry Goods, which was on the first floor of the hotel.

The town was otherwise quiet. Doc nudged the driver to liven the pace, but the wary Feltz did not want to attract attention. They passed into the western reaches of the city where houses grew more sparse; lights from the grand old Swiney mansion on the left perforated the blackness around them. As they approached the bridge over the old Wabash and Erie Canal, the road narrowed. Most of the commercial traffic had long since ceased for the night, but a few oily lamp beams flickered in windows below the gunwales of barges that floated on the mucky water below.

Feltz turned the wagon onto the cemetery road, following the route that Peltier's hearse had taken eight hours earlier. The men stared over shadows of headstones into the empty night, watching and listening for trouble that did not come. By then it was nearly one o'clock; they proceeded to the gate where they sat in brief silence. Then one of the students in the back let out a long whistle, the signal that they were there—and ready.

CHAPTER 9

The Sexton's Mark

JUST BEFORE SUNSET on Thursday, November 22, 1877, the Fort Wayne undertakers, Louis Peltier and Son, had lowered the coffin of Charles Wright, "the well known gardener," into the lawn of Lindenwood Cemetery. Wright's repose would be short. By morning, parts of his dismembered body would be already dispersed between the furnace of the medical college and the roots of a nearby tree.

Earlier that night, around ten o'clock, the disheveled old resurrectionist had poked his apprentice who had, with a routine rehearsed in his recent training, arranged their implements in a long canvas sack, which doubled as a body bag. First into the toolkit went the five-foot-long iron bar that barely fit. Next went a shovel, a rake, an auger, and two tarps. The old man had warned the boy to wrap the metal tools in canvas tarps to keep them from clanking together. There could be no unnecessary noise. The boy then retrieved a dark lantern, whose beam could be squelched by rotating a metal shutter. Because there could be no unnecessary light, either.

Topping up the lantern with coal oil, they walked into the dank November night.

The resurrectionist rarely missed a new grave. With the resumption of classes at the medical college, few funerals—whether they were "fine" ones for the rich or "county" for the poor—escaped his ministrations. Establishment of the school in Fort Wayne the year before had made his job easier by providing a perfect local outlet for his business, with no need to arrange shipping or transportation. The greater the enrollment of students in the college, the more "subjects" were needed for teaching anatomy, and the more daring their procurement became. That November, however, Fort Wayne citizens were on edge. The papers had been running daily stories about Whitey Dan, a tramp whose body had been discovered in a reeking trunk on the depot dock, destined for Michigan, no doubt destined for a medical college.[25]

But despite the public alert, the resurrectionist wasn't going to pass up an opportunity for another snatch, and this one had been arranged in advance. The students weren't picky, but if they didn't want a particular parcel, he could usually find a buyer for it in Ohio or Michigan. He could throw it in a barrel, labeled as whiskey or pickles, or he could stuff it in an old steamer trunk, like Whitey Dan had been. Business was good, but under any circumstances, the trade in human corpses was not for the timid.

The apprentice slung the canvas bag over his shoulder, and the two hiked east toward Washington Street before cutting over to Main. The drizzle had turned icy, which thankfully warded off all but the most ardent late night revelers. The pair moved the mile or so down the dark road, over the Saint Mary's Bridge, and then over the canal toward the graveyard. Resurrectionists knew most of the cemeteries in the county, especially in the dark. He and his apprentice had been to Emanuel Lutheran just a few nights earlier. Although it was a bit farther away than the others, Lindenwood was one of the easiest because it lay sprawled on the western edge of town, a more rural district where they were less likely to draw attention.

---

25 *Fort Wayne Daily Sentinel*, Nov. 28, 1877.

The dark lantern smelled of hot coal oil. He kept it closed. Eyes long adapted to the shadows guided them along the footpath. By 11:30 p.m., they could perceive, outlined against the pitch black of night, the stone gazebos and pergolas that Lindenwood's Superintendent Doswell had arranged throughout the landscape. They made their way along the iron fence, the apprentice counting off the pickets as they passed. No one seemed to be around, but they kept their silence anyway, stepping as quietly as possible. The apprentice knew better than to ask questions; he would learn his macabre trade by watching, listening, and laboring.

The rain, and Charles Wright's funeral procession, had softened the leaves underfoot into compliant silence. They went through the gate, along the stream, and up the hillside among headstones, looking for a newly raked rectangle of earth. The students had said the grave would be about ten steps down the slope from the cemetery's tallest oak. They had no difficulty locating the spot, though the tree was barely blacker than the night sky. No stone was yet in place. The old man grunted; the youth directed the dark lantern's yellow slit toward the lower right corner of the grave, where the dirt was imprinted with the sexton's rune.

When they'd gotten their bearings at the graveside, the youth doused the light, and the older man carefully extracted his implements from the bag. Because of the town's heightened sensitivity to the possibility of their visits, they worked in the dark as much as possible. They knew what they were doing, and the process by now was routine. The resurrectionist probably had worked out his methods back in the 1860s in Ohio where the practice had been, and was still, rampant. He had nearly been caught in Michigan City, Indiana, three years earlier.

Two people typically were required to unearth a body, package it in the sack, and make sure everything looked unscathed in the allotted time. To do it alone was too difficult, especially on nights like that one when damp, clammy fingers made the task harder and longer. But though it was nearly midnight when they reached Wright's graveside, in an hour, the wagon would arrive. They would be warm soon enough.

As deftly as a blind man sets his table, the resurrectionist spread his tools at the head of the grave, arranged so they wouldn't clank together or be left behind in the dark. First came the shovel with which they would dig about a three-foot square hole over the head of the casket. Then came an auger to drill into the lid. Next came the iron bar to pry up the lid and extract the corpse. At last came a rake, to smooth the dirt back over the grave.

As was the custom of their trade, they had brought two, four-by-six-foot canvas tarpaulins, each stained from previous cargo. They spread them carefully along either side of the grave, one to catch the earth, the other to hold the corpse and its trappings. The apprentice rolled the lower end of the left canvas to form a kind of gutter to block stray dirt from running down the hill; he did most of the hard digging, going rapidly at first through the soft and sticky soil, until he'd accumulated a neat mound on the tarpaulin. The old man leaned against the great oak just up the hill, staring into the darkness, alert and wary, ears pricked like a cat awaiting its prey, while the youth worked steadily with the shovel, collecting smaller loads as he went deeper, feeling carefully with the tip.

Finally, the blade scratched the varnished walnut of Charles Wright's coffin. The work slowed as the two men dug together in a practiced ritual of nocturnal precision. Carefully, they softened the earth, first with shovels, then with their hands. Next, they scooped dirt onto the tarp, clearing the head of the coffin and a few inches beyond, down to where its sides began to narrow toward the foot. In twenty minutes, they had cleared enough to get a pry under the lid. The old man then took the auger, pressed its point through the polished surface, into the grain of the wood, and began rotating the handle to bore a one-inch-wide hole. Quickly, he repeated the process a dozen times to pierce the lid with a line of perforations that stretched from one side of the coffin to the other, about two feet below the head. Next they grabbed the forged iron bar, which had a hook on one end, like a shepherd's crook, and a T-bar handle on the other. This was the standard device of the trade, like the blacksmith's hammer or the surgeon's scalpel.

Silently grunting, sweating heavily despite the chill of the night, the resurrectionist advanced the heavy bar until the hook was a couple of inches under the lip of the coffin lid, far enough in to gain some leverage. The nails began to creak and loosen. Both men gripped the T-bar and, with all their weight, levered the shaft toward the ground. The top cracked, then broke, along the row of holes. The men slumped to the leaf-strewn ground and sat silently in the dampness for a minute or so, catching their breath. The loudest, most dangerous part of the process seemed to have transpired without a hitch. The old man cursed and hacked as quietly as possible. Before long, he thought, he would have to find another line of work or end up like the notorious "old Cunny" in Cincinnati.

The drayman William Cunningham, known to the Cincinnati locals as "Old Cunny," had been the most daring and notorious body snatcher of the day. He had supplied bodies to medical colleges all over the Midwest from 1855 to 1871. His methods were brazen. He would dress a body in street clothes, seat it beside him on his wagon, and drive through town in broad daylight to get a delivery to the dissectors. If someone noticed the peculiar posture of his companion, he would slap it in the face, chastising the unfortunate for being drunk in midday. On one occasion, the local constabulary interrupted his midnight resurrection just as two bodies were being slipped from their graves. The police took Cunny to the station and returned the bodies to the funeral home for reburial. Cunny posted bail, and, in the morning, dressed as a bereaved relative and went to the funeral home to claim the bodies, which he promptly delivered to the medical college, only a few hours late. As Cunny aged, he became no less daring, but less adroit in avoiding discovery. His final arrest led to a prison term, during which he fell terminally ill. His fate was just. The local hospital, undoubtedly aware of its nefarious patient, delivered Cunny's dead body to his former patrons at the Medical College of Ohio for anatomic dissection. His skeleton hung in their anatomic museum for many years.[26]

But now, as the resurrectionist and his apprentice continued their work, the clouds seemed to be clearing off; they feared that the half moon peeking through the gloom might soon spoil their cover. They reinserted the hook end of the iron shaft under the shrouded corpse in the now-open coffin; the old man knelt at the graveside and moved his grip toward the hook, snarling at the youth to support the T-bar end. Then he guided the hook with his right hand while groping around the box with his left until he found Wright's head. He turned the bar to engage the dead man's chin with the hook so it wouldn't slip. Next, the diggers gave the corpse a steady heave by the shoulders to shift it toward the coffin's edge. Then they firmly pulled on the T-bar, and the body of Charles Wright rose from its sarcophagus. (*See Fig. 6.*)

Long practice had seared into the resurrectionist's muscle memory the exact tension required to withdraw the body without damaging the head. His waiting customers, who would by then be clomping toward Lindenwood in Fletcher's wagon, would expect their merchandise to be in one piece.

With ritual alacrity, he grasped the body's legs and feet; his apprentice lifted the upper torso. They plopped Charles Wright onto his tarpaulin. In a few moments, Wright was stripped— shoes, pants, shirt, tie, coat, and undergarments were slipped off and neatly piled. Wright's nakedness exposed the ravages of his disease. He hadn't been able to eat a decent meal for weeks before he died. Wasting of his body allowed his gold ring to slip off more

---

26 Linden F. Edwards, *Cincinnati's "Old Cunny" A Notorious Purveyor of Human Flesh* (Public Library of Fort Wayne and Allen County, 1955).

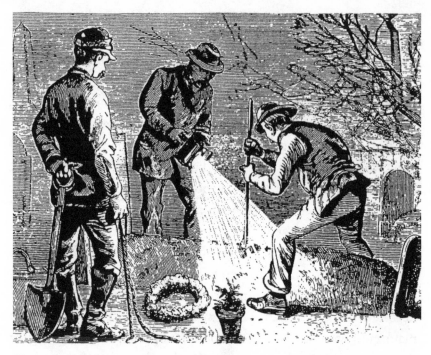

Figure 6. Resurrectionists at Work. At left, an assistant holds a shovel and the resurrectionist's bar with the hook on the end; the man in the middle holds the dark lantern while the old man bores with the auger into the coffin lid. Reproduced from the Indiana Medical History Quarterly with permission of the Indiana State Historical Society.

easily. The resurrectionist reluctantly tossed the ring back into the coffin with the rest of Wright's clothes and belongings. Tempting as it was, stealing the sepulchral accoutrements simply was not worth the risk. Body snatching was one thing, a misdemeanor that carried a fine, but the robbing of property, even a corpse's property, was a felony that could result in a trip to prison. Technically, the body itself was not property, but the clothing and jewelry, even the shroud, were part of the estate and therefore belonged to the descendants. Besides, the old man was a professional, and his customers had contracted for a corpse, nothing else.

The apprentice quickly pulled the sack over Wright's naked body, pursing the ties around the revolting head. The older man heaved the sack over his shoulder, folding the stiffened Wright at the waist. He trudged a hundred feet down the slope to the roadside along the creek where he crouched well back into the dark among the trees, the sack on the ground beside him. He thought he could hear the distant hoofbeats of Fletcher's approaching dray horse. It was nearly one o'clock.

The apprentice stayed behind to finish up the details. He opened the dark lantern to survey the area for missed items and just as quickly doused it again. In the dark, he scrunched the coffin lid down, ignoring the splintered wood along the fracture edge, which, it was hoped, no one would ever see. He replaced the dirt, slightly overfilling the hole, then raking the surface as smooth as he could get it. He rolled up the tool kit and moved off to join his companion. About halfway down the hill, he stopped short, remembering something—and wouldn't the old codger take it out of his hide if he'd forgotten? He quickly lay down the tools and ran back to kneel by the lower corner of Wright's grave. Hastily, he replicated the sexton's signature mark in the freshly raked soil. The rune looked a little crooked, not quite right, but the hour was late, so it would have to do. He raced for the road.

Undertakers and cemeteries went to great lengths to protect the graves for their customers who were only too aware of the threat of body theft. One strategy was for cemeteries to build an enclosed and heavily secured "death house" where the body would be stored and allowed to putrefy for several days before burial, rendering it useless to the dissectors. In the abstract, the "death house" seemed to be the most effective deterrent, but the idea of a loved one's earthly remains rotting away in a shed, elaborately constructed though it might be, repelled the average mourner. After Wright's resurrection, some civic leaders called for construction of a death house in Fort Wayne, but the concept proved too gruesome to be accepted.[27] The special cast iron coffins—some with explosive

---

27 *Fort Wayne Daily News*, November 27, 1877, 2.

lids—that were being developed, were resulting in logistics and expense that often outweighed the horror of the potential body snatching. A less expensive deterrent was to lay a heavy, sometimes ornately cast, iron plate over the buried casket to impede its possible disturbance, but this was proving a mere inconvenience to the resurrectionists. Today, those shield-like plates can sometimes be seen in old cemeteries, rising, rusted and disintegrating, to the surface of the soil like a tree root breaking through the grass.

Cemeteries also could arrange to install a special wrought iron fence around the grave, but this seemed like more of a gesture than a real impediment. (*See Fig. 7.*) After all, the fence could only be constructed in advance or be erected after it was too late for the body to be attractive to resurrectionists. As it was, if no immediate

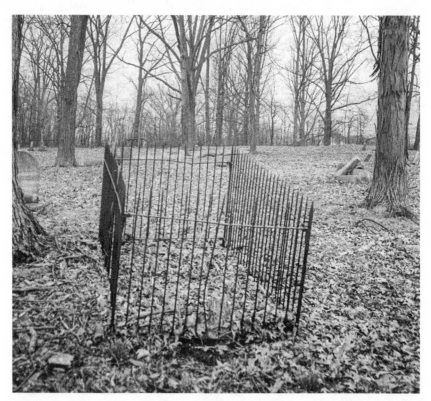

Figure 7. An iron fence encircling a gravesite in Roanoke, Indiana. Photographed by the author.

buyer was available after resurrections, the bodies had to be packed in barrels of vinegar, brine, or whiskey to prolong their suitability. In those cases, once a customer was found, intemperate medical students extracted the grisly insoluble. Chronically short of funds for their scant leisure time, the students often drained off and then drank the foul liquor that remained in the barrel, which they christened "rotgut whiskey."

In theory, the common method to protect the grave was for the sexton to place a special mark, unique to him or to his cemetery, on the soil. As was done in Wright's case, it was often contrived, by using the shovel or rake, into a geometric pattern similar to a brand for ranch cattle. In other cases, small stones, twigs, or personal objects would be arranged in a unique pattern that would be difficult to replicate. If the mark remained undisturbed through the night, the sexton could then reassure the family that the grave was safe. In actual practice, the sexton of the cemetery often had a financial arrangement with the local resurrectionists whereby he would lead them to the grave, stand as a sentinel during the exhumation and, afterward, replace the crucial mark. One story tells of a giant of a gravedigger with the largest feet in town. After the funeral, he would imprint his great boot print into the newly raked soil and reassure the widow that, if the boot mark was still there in the morning, she would know the grave had not been disturbed. He would then lead the grave robbers to the site, help them dig up the body, and carefully replace his great boot print upon the soil.

But now, as the hour of assignation approached, all seemed fine with the Charles Wright snatching; the resurrectionist clearly heard the steady clip of a horse and wagon proceeding along the roadway. When it stopped, he could make out the men on the seat in front (one looked like a doctor he'd worked for before) and two others crouched in the back. A moment later, he heard the long, low whistle from the darkness over the trees. Then came the footsteps: the doctor and two younger men stepped into the muted moonlight along the path.

The resurrectionist and his apprentice moved quietly toward the wagon and loaded the cadaver. The two students jumped onto the wagon bed and, with the third student who had remained crouched in the back, slipped the grisly corpse from the sack and returned the sack to the old man. The doctor paid the resurrectionist, who stuffed the bills into his pocket, dumped the tarp-wrapped tools into the sack and, with his apprentice, disappeared into the darkness. They were never seen, identified, or heard of again.

As A.E. resumed his seat next to the wagon driver, the students in the back wrapped the body of Charles Wright in the old blankets they'd brought, as if to warm him from the morning chill.

Meanwhile, the wagon driver, Charles Feltz, kept his eyes focused ahead. When he heard the signal that the students were done with their task, he clucked his guttural grunt and pulled the left rein to turn the horse back onto the road. The wheels grated on the gravel; they retraced their tracks, crossing over the old Wabash and Erie Canal and heading directly to the medical college on Broadway and Washington.

Feltz did not speak a word. He did not look back toward his load. He worked for Mr. Fletcher and Mr. Powers, and they'd been hired to provide a wagon and driver. It was their wagon, and he drove it. As far as he was concerned, he had picked up a load of merchandise. He had not asked about the contents; the clients had not explained. It could as well have been a sack of potatoes— whatever it was, was Fletcher's business, not his. Occasionally the doctor on the seat beside him made a comment, but Feltz just nodded. Then they emerged onto Main Street, heading east toward the town. Charles Feltz's passengers seemed to pulsate with anticipation. But he only wanted to drop off his passengers and their suspicious load so he could return the wagon and forget about it. Maybe he could grab some sleep.

The wagon passed the now-quiet Anderson's Hotel on the corner of Broadway and Jefferson Streets; Feltz turned left onto Washington and pulled to a stop alongside Wright's Drug Store. Despite the hour, lights flickered from the school chambers on an upper floor. Smoke drifted from the chimney. It was clear that they were expected. From the seat beside him, the doctor dropped to the ground, walked to the side door on Broadway, and knocked. A young man opened the door. The doctor quickly slipped into the building. The students in the back pulled their blanketed prize from the rear of the wagon, much the way the casket had been slid from Peltier's hearse ten hours before. They followed their professor into the building. And Feltz drove away; his night's work was done; the transaction, completed; the parcel, delivered.

A.E. made his way up the rickety stairs to the third floor laboratory; his students were behind him, struggling under their awkward load. Another student admitted the small group through the heavy door, then locked it behind them. Two overhead gas jets threw a dim glow on the row of makeshift tables in the large room. A blackboard hung from one wall; a cabinet on another wall held shelves of ominous specimen bottles. Suspended from a ceiling hook screwed through its pale caput, an articulated skeleton surveyed the oft run scene of its own dismemberment playing again and again before its empty orbs. One of the tables, which had been cobbled together from wide planks and two sawhorses, held a corpse in an advanced stage of disarticulation. (*See Fig. 8.*) Chewing tobacco, a prophylactic against the smell, bulged the cheeks of student dissectors as they hunched over their specimen with dissection knives and bone saws. A bucket beneath the table held the detritus of their day's work. A roaring fire burned in the furnace both for warmth and to serve as a receptacle for the unwanted *disjecta membra*.

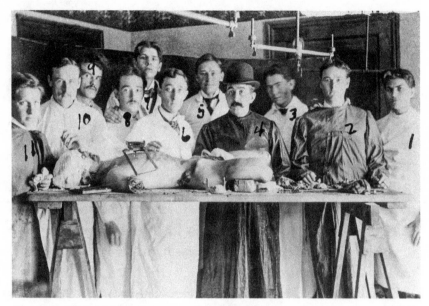

Figure 8. Dissection Laboratory, Fort Wayne College of Medicine, ca. 1897. Reproduced with the permission of the Allen County-Fort Wayne Historical Society.

The students hauled the awkward bundle and staggered to a table that had been cleared in anticipation of the delivery. Then they unceremoniously dumped Charles Wright's body onto the wood planks. The soiled shroud of their professor's old blankets slid from the cadaver and revealed its withered form. Like an actor past his prime, the demonstrator of anatomy stepped from the darkness of his corner desk into the light cast by the overhead lamp. He had wrapped himself in an old cloak that was indelibly mottled with the stains of past performances. As was typical, five students in all gathered around him while he proceeded to perform a cursory examination of the new arrival.

Wright's head was covered with abscesses, now dried and congealed but ominously distinct. The body, though emaciated, was intact and usable, even informative, but the dissectors would need to work quickly. Remembering too well Professor Myers's admonition of two nights before about the need for anonymity of the cadaver, the demonstrator directed one of his students to retrieve a long, steel-bladed dissection knife and a bone saw from the cabinet at the end of the capacious room. The knife blade shimmered blue in the amber light of the student lamp that had been set up near the table. The body had been placed in the supine position, on its back, as if Wright's sightless eyes might catch one final glimpse of his tormentors. Deftly, the demonstrator cut through Charles's neck with the knife—through the skin, the windpipe, the jugular, and carotid vessels, slicing through scrofulous glands that no longer resisted. Quickly, he exchanged the blade for the saw; the bone fell away easily. The last remnants of skin at the neck were severed. One of the students held open an old flour sack within which Charles Wright's head was deposited for its final disposition, which would be burial under a nearby tree.

Following his professor's mumbled directions, the student unlatched the door and, with the flour sack tightly in hand, disappeared down the stairs. He returned half an hour later without his burden and resumed his position at the table holding the torso of Charles Wright.

The demonstrator gave his last instructions for the night: what and where to cut, and where to read in *Gray's Anatomy*. The students seemed to have the dissection well in hand; it was, after all, the second procedure that week. Near his seat in the darkened corner, the exhausted Aaron Elliott Van Buskirk, newly appointed, recently reprimanded, demonstrator of anatomy, replaced the soiled smock that he wore for dissections on a coat hook. He retrieved his tall black hat and the long black coat for which he would become known. He slipped out the door, down the stairs, tired but content in the perception that he had fulfilled the duties of his position.

It was by then around three o'clock Friday morning. The rain had stopped; the clouds had cleared. In the waning moonlight, A.E. walked contentedly toward his home on Locust Street. He knew that, over the course of the next several nights, Charles Wright would be slowly but inexorably disassembled for their edification, satisfying both the students' needs for firsthand experience and the demands of the senior faculty. After all, two cadavers in one week should go a long way toward pleasing his superiors. He hoped to catch a few hours of sleep before dawn.

CHAPTER 10

Doswell's Disturbance

O
N THE MORNING OF Friday, November 23, 1877, John Doswell arose early after a restless night. Doswell was worried. As superintendent of Lindenwood Cemetery, he considered himself fortunate to have been spared most of the scandalous disturbances in graveyards that were plaguing other cemeteries in town, but he knew it was probably only a matter of time. Well versed in the body snatching lore of his native England, Doswell had developed his own "sexton's mark" years earlier. Either he or his trusted sexton always personally placed their mark upon the soil, their pledge that an intact mark in the morning meant the sepulcher was safe. The sexton had left his mark clearly visible on Wright's grave.

The community of Fort Wayne bestowed a particular pride upon Lindenwood Cemetery because the people viewed it as much a place for bucolic leisure as for mourning their dead. Couples often strolled among the trees, and even picnicked on warm days in the stone gazebo's cool shade, away from the bustle of the town center. The new, tall, wrought iron fence lent both a reassuring austerity and a formidable barrier for any nefarious souls who might be contemplating a midnight dig. Unless the local college had ordered a specific body, the resurrectionists usually left Lindenwood alone. Its large size and popularity, in addition to the inconvenience of having to trek out from town, usually diverted the resurrectionists' attention to the smaller, more accessible graveyards. But since the medical college had re-opened in the fall, despite the precautions of the staff and the barriers around the burial sites and the grounds, no grave was really safe.

Because Lindenwood Cemetery's president, Isaac De Groff Nelson was also on the medical college's board of directors, Doswell knew that the school was pressed for suitable subjects. He also knew, for certain, that the body snatchers had been steadily at work around town—their machinations had been regularly reported in the daily newspapers since the beginning of the academic year. On October 2, 1877, the *Fort Wayne Daily Sentinel* observed that while twenty-five students attended the medical school, the "ghouls" were again working the cemeteries. Either to reassure the skeptics or warn the mourners, a week later the paper reported that the medical school was flourishing. On October 16, the *Sentinel* observed that "four stiffs ornament the dissecting rooms on Broadway." The papers also noted a rumor that, during the preceding week, a body had been stolen from the Catholic Cemetery. By the time of Charles Wright's funeral a month later, the papers were running a commentary almost daily about the body of the murdered tramp, "Whitey Dan," that Professor Myers had tried to divert, unsuccessfully, to the school for dissection. Aside from specific orders from the medical college, the professional body snatchers took just about any body they could snatch but, for unclaimed material, they usually found it safer to ship the body out of state.

With unwonted anxiety, John Doswell dressed quickly and took only a few bites of his breakfast before leaving the house. By the feeble glow of the autumnal dawn, Doswell rode directly to Lindenwood, intending to bypass his office and headed immediately toward Wright's gravesite on the gentle hillside. He vainly hoped that any peculiar disorder and compression of the leaves in the surrounding area could be attributed to the funeral crowd of the previous afternoon. But when he reached the cemetery gate, his premonitions validated his worst fears: tracks from a turning wagon had left their spoor in the gravel.

Doswell hitched his buggy along the roadway at the base of the slope, closer to the graves than where the wagon had stopped the night before. Up the gentle slope among the limestone headstones, his premonition grew more ominous. The surface soil didn't look right, as if it had been re-raked. And the sexton's mark had been subtly, but definitely, disturbed, crooked, as if hastily contrived.

Staring at the roughened soil, Doswell contemplated his choices. None were appealing, for none would reflect well upon him. There could be no denying that the grave had been disturbed, probably its contents removed. Mr. Isaac De Groff Nelson himself had been worried about the possibility of a grave robbery and undoubtedly would arrive soon to make his own inspection. Nelson had attended the funeral and warned Doswell and the sexton to be on the alert for trouble. The latter assured them that all would be well. Doswell might have considered an attempt to rake over the soil and replace the mark exactly, but it was not worth the risk in broad daylight. Soon, the family would also examine the grave for any alterations in the imprint. Doswell knew he had to report the incident immediately so proper steps could be taken; an exhumation would need to be arranged to confirm whether or not the grave had been opened.

With little doubt in his mind about what they would find, John Doswell, superintendent of Lindenwood Cemetery, trudged back down the hill and ascended his buggy once more. He turned the horse and followed the route that, only hours earlier, Feltz's wagon had taken into town.

Doswell drove directly into the city to speak with Lindenwood's president, Mr. Nelson. Isaac De Groff Nelson received the news with equanimity of his years and stature: he was not particularly surprised. As a member of the board of directors of both the medical college and the cemetery, he was well aware of the internecine struggles within the former and naturally concerned for the latter. He was, however, annoyed that his staff had let him down. He would arrange for Wright's grave to be opened immediately, and he would assemble the board of trustees as soon as possible. Louis Peltier would inform the family.

Nelson had been president of Lindenwood Cemetery since its inception; the leaders of Fort Wayne, including the august Hugh McCulloch, comprised its board of trustees. Nelson called for an emergency meeting to convene the following morning. They needed to discuss the situation and develop a plan of action. Louis Peltier was terribly upset by the news and favored contacting the Wright family immediately. It was by no means the first time Peltier had dealt with a theft of one of his newly buried bodies, but he had not expected the sanctity of Lindenwood to be violated. Peltier took Doswell with him to confront the unenviable task of explaining to Mary Wright what had happened.

In the abstract, their news should come as no surprise, because at that time and place, it was every widow's fear. But the reality might be difficult to accept, that Mary's husband's body lay not in eternal rest, but stolen, tossed about like a sack of produce and probably already dismembered for the students' academic scrutiny. She had known about body snatching and had, after all, discussed protective measures with Mr. Peltier. In the final analysis, they had convinced her that the burial at Lindenwood would provide some measure of protection, and that the grave would be watched. They had explained about the mark. They expressed their fantasy that most snatches occurred in the potter's field, not at places like Lindenwood. It was true that potter's fields were the ghouls' preference; those places were usually less guarded, less scrutinized in a darkened, neglected corner of a graveyard. The students didn't care about the social standing of the body; for their purposes, one was as good as another, so long as it was intact with all its parts.

Wearing their discomfiture like the mourner's armband, Doswell and Peltier knocked on Mary Wright's door. Charlotte and her husband, John Christie, who had spent the night with her mother, Mary, listened with horror and smoldering anger. Together, the Wright family, Peltier, and Doswell returned to Lindenwood not twenty-four hours after they had thrown the first dirt on Charles's coffin.

In a short time, Doswell rousted the sexton with instructions to gather his tools. Without a word, they all gathered at the gravesite. The sexton began to dig. It only took a few shovels to lend full credence to their worst suspicions: fresh splinters of wood speckled the soft black Indiana soil; when they reached the surface of the casket, they could see that the lid had been fractured from side to side. Lifting the fragment, they found no body, just the shroud and the clothes that had belonged to Charles Wright.

Doswell immediately summoned the police, as well as the Lindenwood Board of Trustees, each of whom Nelson had already contacted about a meeting to be held as soon as possible.

After the Lindenwood Board of Trustees' emergency meeting on Saturday, the headline in the *Daily Sentinel* blared, "A Grave Robbed. Lindenwood Cemetery visited by Human Hyenas." The issue reported that, from the cemetery office on the morning of Saturday, November 24, 1877, the Trustees adopted resolutions that condemned the affair and offered for any person providing evidence leading to detection and conviction of the perpetrators the following resolution and a $1,000 award: Resolution:

> WHEREAS, It has come to the knowledge of this Board that the body of Charles Wright, a respectable citizen of this place, having a family, who was buried in the ground of this corporation of the 22nd last, was stolen from the grave on the same night by a person or persons unknown to this Board; and,

WHEREAS, Said burial grounds have been desecrated by a most wanton act in violation of public morals, decency, and the law of the land, it is hereby

ORDERED, That a reward be offered by the Board of $1,000 to be paid to the person or persons giving such information as will lead to the detection and conviction of any of the parties engaged in the act. It's further

RESOLVED, that this order be made public, and that all good citizens be requested to aid in bringing these criminals to justice.

I.D.G. Nelson, Pres. J.D. Bond, Sec.[28]

Later that afternoon, a police officer, apparently one of those who had investigated the medical college, emboldened himself to apply for the award on the grounds that he had "recovered" the body, though it was by then dismembered and partially dissected at the school. The Lindenwood Board of Trustees met for a second time that same day, that time at the Fort Wayne National Bank, to address the officer's application. The board clarified its position that the award would be delivered only when the perpetrators were both apprehended and convicted, not simply for recovery of the body. In fact, the policeman had only observed some cadavers on the tables in the school but none were specifically identifiable as Wright. What they did not know was that, by then, parts of the gardener's corpse had already been burned in the furnace, and the telltale head buried under a nearby tree.

News of the $1,000 award spread quickly. The Monday papers reported that detectives from Chicago, Cincinnati, and Buffalo had arrived in Fort Wayne and were questioning citizens about what had happened. Pinkerton men staked out the medical college and

---

28 *Fort Wayne Daily News*, November 24, 1877.

stalked every student and faculty member as they came and went. Despite the application of the brazen police officer, papers of the week of November 26 reported that the exact state and location of the body remained unknown. Some speculated that, like the corpse of Whitey Dan, it had been shipped out of town. Others believed it still lay, somehow hidden, in the chambers of the college. No one doubted that it had been stolen for purposes of dissection. And all eyes were turned toward the medical college on Broadway.

CHAPTER 11

Captain Diehl

LINDENWOOD'S $1,000 OFFER had served its intended purpose. A half-dozen private detectives scoured the streets of Fort Wayne for clues to Wright's resurrection, but they had nothing to show for their efforts. For weeks, the crime went unsolved. No one found the body. Some people speculated that it had been shipped to Ann Arbor to the University of Michigan or to Indianapolis where several medical schools coexisted. The Fort Wayne school spouted its rote mantra that they acquired their subjects from Chicago. Pat Conover, a reporter for the *Fort Wayne Sentinel,* was so convinced that the perpetrators had exchanged Wright's body for another in Chicago, that he went there to examine the Illinois schools' dissection tables firsthand. He found no trace of Charles Wright. As the hours and days passed, most people believed that the body had been dismembered beyond recognition and would never be found.

Despite the multitude of private interests in solving the crime and reaping the reward, the official responsibility fell upon one man, Police Chief Hugh Diehl. In the atmosphere of scandal, debauchery, and corruption, which had long pervaded the local police force, Chief Diehl had only recently assumed his post. A wounded and decorated veteran of the Civil War, he was an airbrake inspector for the Pennsylvania Railroad, a post to which he would return when his term with the police was over. Widely respected for his levelheaded, workman-like approach, the methodical Diehl was accustomed to pressure and to detection, though of a different sort. Accidents were the railroad's most fearsome and frequent nightmare. The railroad lines relied heavily on the cold, if stolid, acumen of people like Diehl to detect aberrations before they became full-blown catastrophes. Ignoring the widespread furor that permeated Fort Wayne, he assumed personal leadership of the Wright investigation. He needed to solve this crime badly; though he wanted the reward as much as anyone, the possibility of out-detecting the out-of-town experts would lend needed credibility to his department.

Diehl and his officers first inspected the medical school on Washington and Broadway, but, when they attempted to enter the odious dissection room on the third floor, they found its doors locked from within. In the absence of a warrant, the faculty blocked police access to the crucial laboratory. The school officials denied any knowledge of Wright; they patiently explained that all of their subjects had been shipped in from Chicago. By the time police finally gained official entry to the dissection chambers, they found several cadavers lying upon the tables, in various stages of dismemberment, but none were identifiable as Wright. One cadaver, in particular, roused the officers' suspicion because it was headless, but that also meant that there was nothing specific to identify.

By Sunday, the Pinkerton detectives combed the byways of Fort Wayne, quizzing anyone who may have known something that would lead them to the $1,000.[29] Every student, faculty member, and worker at the medical college acquired a second shadow, but to little discernible effect. The detectives knew only too well that body snatches usually went unresolved, even among the few that were actually discovered. Professional resurrectionists were too

---

29 *Fort Wayne Daily News*, November 26, 1877, 1.

accomplished at covering their tracks, and their customers, too adept at discarding the spent bodies.

One reporter from the *Daily News* managed an interview with an anonymous doctor at the medical college who admitted that he had some past experience with body snatching—that nearly every faculty member had. He described the process similar to how it had occurred in Wright's case: digging down to the head of the coffin, breaking through the lid, using a hooked rod to extract the body, "chucking" it into a sack and throwing it into a wagon. Did he believe the snatchers would be caught? "Not unless they are some d-----d fools who don't understand the business."[30]

On Monday, the local newspapers continued to tantalize their readers with hope for a speedy resolution to the crime. Tuesday's paper suggested that the solution might have been near, but most readers didn't really believe it.

The grand jury interviewed anyone and everyone who could possibly have been involved or knowledgeable about the theft of Charles Wright's body from Lindenwood Cemetery. By peculiar coincidence, Mr. Isaac De Groff Nelson—the same Nelson who was president of the Lindenwood Cemetery and founding director of the college of medicine—also served as foreman of the grand jury, but his personal interest did not seem to accelerate the investigation's progress.

A week after Wright's death, the papers complained impatiently that the grave robbers remained free and unknown.

By the first of the second week after Wright's resurrection, the grand jury had subpoenaed and interviewed each medical student and faculty member, one by one. They completed the process by Saturday, December 8, but had little to show for their work. Three days later, even the most optimistic of the newspapers bemoaned the lack of progress.

---

30 *Fort Wayne Daily News*, November 26, 1877.

The grand jury investigation, however, did confirm the common public impression that the disruption of Wright's grave was by no means an isolated incident. Apparently body snatches were taking place regularly and continually because the medical college was in continual need of cadavers. But no specific details were forthcoming. Reports of many of the snatchings had appeared in the local papers. The shocking aspect of the Wright case was not that it had transpired, but that it had occurred at the city's own Lindenwood, a place that many considered too inviolable for body snatchers to risk apprehension. To compound the affront, Charles Wright had been a well-known citizen of Fort Wayne.

Curiously, on Tuesday, December 11, Mr. Sullivan, the sexton of the Catholic Cemetery, reported that he had been awakened during the previous night by the persistent barking of a dog. He claimed to have arisen from his bed and had followed the dog into the graveyard where he interrupted two men at work. Sullivan alleged that the men had recoiled and quickly ran off. He investigated and found the half-filled grave of Mrs. Mary Neidhofer who actually had died some three weeks earlier, on November 20. She had been buried in the morning of the same day as Charles Wright. Mr. Peltier, the undertaker, was called to investigate; he found the coffin empty. The story was suspicious because any professional body snatcher would have known that after three weeks the body would have decomposed beyond any utility for dissection. Most likely, the body had been stolen long before, probably the same night as Wright's. Although nothing further was reported of this case, its belated exposure may well have been staged to divert public attention from the Wright case.

The tragic accidental death of Mary Neidhofer, the young mother of three small children, had been broadly covered in the local papers.[31] The discovery that her body had also been stolen would serve as a handy distraction to pull the white heat of public

---

31 *Fort Wayne Daily News*, December 13, 1877.

scrutiny off the Wright case. Instead, the charade only heightened the general sense of communal indignation that permeated Fort Wayne as its residents prepared for their Christmas holidays.

But, undaunted by the intense surveillance of local graveyards, the resurrectionists continued to ply their trade. On Friday, December 21, another snatch was discovered, that time in neighboring Monroeville, Dr. Van Buskirk's hometown. The day before, the dead body of a tramp named Bearkett had been discovered about six miles west of town. His remains were taken to the local cemetery and buried at public expense. A group of concerned local volunteers agreed to stand watch over the grave for six days and nights to prevent it from being disturbed. Several people were appointed to guard the grave each night, but the body was stolen anyway. Neither the corpse nor the perpetrators were ever found.

By the middle of December, the out-of-town detectives had given up their quest for the $1,000 reward and gone home, but Hugh Diehl soldiered on. It was his job. Chief Diehl was the first to admit that he wanted the money, but, even with his familiarity with the principals and the territory, he, too was having a difficult time. The medicos were not helping. They made no effort to cooperate with the investigation of the Wright case: they fabricated outrageous and inconsistent stories designed primarily to shift attention off themselves. Many of the doctors had their own agendas, formed well before the discovery of Wright's exhumation. In general, the Fort Wayne doctors were a pretty rough-and-ready lot who worked hard to preserve their own position in the community. Many of the older physicians had begun their practices as apprentices on the old Indiana frontier. They were not about to jeopardize their hard-earned community status for something as mundane as a body snatch.

Medicine of the 1870s attracted a raw sort of individual, always ready for a fight, verbal or otherwise. Doctors were often men without much formal education, and were more accustomed to histrionics than reasoned discourse. Like many trades, one could take up doctoring as an apprentice and eventually hang up one's own shingle. With a successful practice and a few fortuitous cures, a young doctor could achieve the professional status of a lawyer or preacher. For a bright young man with more in his head than in his pocket, medicine could offer the shortest route to community stature and even to a modicum of wealth.

By late November 1877, antipathy toward doctors in general, and toward the medical college in particular, coursed mightily throughout the city of Fort Wayne. People simply didn't trust them. The fact that the local newspapers regularly criticized the local physicians intimated that the mortality of the sick was unusually high. People could not help but wonder that, if the medical college was supposed to have attracted such great doctors, why were so many people dying in Fort Wayne? To make matters worse, the resumption of the medical college classes had signaled more than the coming of autumn, and the citizens of Fort Wayne soon not only feared for their lives at the hands of the doctors, but also for the fate of their dead. The papers commented that "... ghouls have again been working in the cemeteries," and again, "The fall trade is opening well—especially with doctors and undertakers."

Amid the criticism for their collective ineptitude, miserliness, and desecrations of the local graveyards, many of the local physicians, both college faculty and other practitioners in the community, were called upon to testify in a court case that became a portent for the coming months. A man named Hamilton stood trial for raping a woman named Catherine Warstler. The court summoned many of the Fort Wayne doctors to testify. Dr. Harold A. Clark, the newly appointed professor of anatomy, gave indirect evidence about other rape cases he had encountered. Next, Dr. Thomas Jefferson Dills was called, but he demanded that he be compensated for his time before he would discuss the case. The judge held Dills in contempt and jailed him until he agreed to speak before the court. Another prominent physician, Dr. A.P. Buchman, also refused to testify and joined Dills in the dungeon. Then, the controversial Dr. William H.

Myers strode to the stand and stated that although he sympathized with the sentiments of Dills, he agreed to tell the court what he knew.

As Dills and Buchman granted interviews from their cells, the jailed doctors became subjects of ridicule for some, but martyrs to the cause of many physicians. Even the state medical society in Indianapolis took up the matter of whether or not a physician should be paid to render their opinion before the court, and about half of its members came down in favor. The issue would eventually wind its way through the courts and finally, six months later, to the Indiana State Supreme Court. In the meantime, the freely given testimony of Professors Clark and Myers further inflamed the already incendiary conditions among the local physicians and in the community at large.

The final two months of 1877 had forged a situation at the college from which it could scarcely recover. From its inception, the medical college had arisen within in a culture of dissension both internally, among members of the faculty, and externally, in competition with other community doctors. The *Sentinel* contended that there was ". . . more undeveloped medical skill to the square foot in Fort Wayne than any other city in the state."[32] Meanwhile, the medical students pressed their instructors for more cadavers. The faculty, in turn, exhorted their colleagues in the anatomy department, Professor Clark and Demonstrator Van Buskirk, to be more productive. Neither were experienced anatomists. Van Buskirk had just completed his medical degree the year before taking his post at the medical college, and Clark had been a professor of chemistry, not anatomy. Perhaps the faculty doubted their qualifications; surely, many of the professors questioned the vigor with which their anatomists contracted for dissection material. As early as November 7, the local papers had rumored that changes in the medical college administration were in the offing. In addition,

---

32 *Fort Wayne Daily Sentinel*, November 29, 1877.

the doctors themselves were unhappy about the state of the school. Many of A.E.'s colleagues fumed at the influential Professor Myers for not standing by Dills and Buchman.

William Herschel Myers, one of Fort Wayne's most prominent physicians and, by some accounts, her first surgeon, seemed to stir controversy wherever he went, relishing the limelight, favorable or not. By giving free testimony in the Hamilton case, Myers and Clark had broken ranks with the other doctors, and had facilitated the martyrdom of Drs. Dills and Buchman who continued to sulk in the local jail. The school became divided over these and other issues. The desecration of the popular Charles Wright's grave and the intense investigation that followed further polarized the faculty.

Antagonists to Myers and Clark began to hold secret meetings in hopes of expelling them from the college faculty. In contrast, the medical students reserved their highest esteem for Professor Myers, for his clinical skill and, especially, for his devotion to furthering their medical education. None of the faculty was more assiduous in paying attention to the students' needs, especially in the clinics of St. Joseph Hospital where the medical school maintained a teaching service for the poor. There the faculty supervised medical students in their care of the city's indigent residents. Even in the midst of the internecine rancor and community attention, the unabashed Professor Myers never missed his teaching assignments. Most of the students, oblivious to the sociopolitical aspects of the affair, sided with their mentor.

As previously mentioned, Myers, amidst the Wright furor, disdained community sensitivity about the dissection business by attempting to direct yet another body, that of the murdered tramp, Whitey Dan, to the college for the students' dissection. After having been discovered in an old trunk at the railroad depot, Whitey Dan's body had been taken to the hospital where Dr. Myers was scheduled to perform an autopsy. Instead, Myers tried to move the body to the medical college for the students' ministrations in their anatomy laboratory. St. Joseph Hospital considered his attempt an egregious breach of its agreement with the medical school. On December 2, the hospital's executive committee, led by Bishop J. Dwenger, interrupted one of Professor Myers's lectures to confront him with their umbrage over liberties he had taken with hospital patients. The class was prematurely dismissed, and Bishop Dwenger demanded both that Professor Myers and his colleague, Dr. Clark, withdraw from the faculty of the college and be excluded from the hospital. The following day, St. Joseph Hospital closed its clinics for the medical school and gave the college ten days to vacate the hospital facilities. In a separate action, they expelled both Dr. Myers and Dr. Clark from the St. Joseph Hospital medical staff, an action that would prevent the doctors from being able to admit their patients.

In reality, that incident provided the ideal opportunity that many of the college faculty needed to address their grievances with Professors Myers and Clark. Hoping to restore its relationship with the hospital and to solve its internal struggles with the same stroke of the pen, the college faculty drew up a petition demanding that Clark and Myers resign their professorships, but the professors had already beaten them to the draw. The petition was never presented because Myers and Clark had successfully persuaded the superior court to grant an injunction that restrained the faculty from holding a meeting to discuss their fate. In a separate action, the court also issued a restraining order against St. Joseph Hospital that prevented its planned expulsion of Drs. Myers and Clark.

These squabbles among the doctors had no direct bearing upon the body snatch case, but they worked to Chief Diehl's favor. The doctors had, by that time, abandoned all pretense of loyalty to each other. Each scrambled to fend for himself. On Tuesday, December 18, the daily papers reported that the police were closing in. By then, they had interviewed all the doctors, each of whom was becoming increasingly nervous, anxious to shift blame to anyone else. The infamous Harold Clark and William Myers, who were having their own struggles with the local hospital, their faculty colleagues, and even the local medical society, finally agreed to testify against the perpetrators.

Shortly thereafter, by apparent coincidence, Diehl happened upon the proverbial street corner where he "serendipitously" overheard the two doctors, Myers and Clark, discussing the Wright affair. In the course of their conversation, Diehl heard them reveal the name of one of the grave robbers.

CHAPTER 12

Nolle Prosequi

AUTHOR'S NOTE: The three trials reported daily in the Fort Wayne papers were nearly exact transcripts of testimony along with editorial comments. The material in Chapters 12, 13, and 14 has been derived from those transcripts.

ARON AND MARY JANE VAN BUSKIRK weren't having much of a Christmas holiday. A.E. was shadowed day and night; his colleagues avoided his company. As the most junior member of the faculty and the demonstrator of anatomy to boot, he was the most obvious in line to take the charge. On Thursday, December 27, A.E. arose early. Just as the winter sun broke over the Maumee River, he arrived at the medical college on the corner of Broadway and Washington Streets. Sensing that he would be preoccupied with more urgent matters later in the day, the demonstrator went directly to the anatomical laboratory to prepare for the day's dissection.

Around nine o'clock, he heard footsteps clamoring up the rear stairs followed by a great commotion in the hall outside the laboratory; men were shouting and banging on the chamber's heavy door. A.E. sighed in resignation as he opened the door and admitted Police Chief Diehl and his uniformed associates into the room.

The police presented a warrant to the anatomist for his arrest on the charge of stealing the body of Charles Wright from its new grave during the night of November 22. Glad that he had arrived early enough to set up the laboratory for the day's work, Van Buskirk went quietly. The police led him down Broadway to the nearby offices of G. William Sommers, a medical student who was also a pharmacist. They arrested him, too. In time for the afternoon newspaper editions to get their breaking news, the police chief then marched his prisoners down Berry Street. When they reached the corner of Berry and Calhoun in the center of town, they had to wait while the streetcar passed before a small crowd who had gathered to watch the spectacle. The chief then conducted his prisoners across Calhoun to a ramshackle, false-fronted low building that was squeezed between the imposing Aveline Hotel and Pixley's dry goods store. The unprepossessing, white-framed structure housed the modest chambers of Squire Daniel Ryan, justice of the peace. (*See Fig. 9.*) Ryan was expecting them. He had already detained the hack driver, a man named Charles Feltz, from Fletcher and Powers Livery. The afternoon papers blared that Chief Diehl had arrested the medicos with the headline: "Snatching the Snatchers!"[33]

Throughout the month of December, even as the newspapers ran daily accounts of the doings of private detectives and the ineptitude of their local police, Chief Diehl had been quietly gathering evidence and assembling his case. He now revealed that he had had the case in hand all along: a few days after the body had been stolen, he had managed to interview one of Fletcher and Powers's hack drivers, Charles Feltz, who, after intensive interrogation, reluctantly admitted (probably in exchange for the immunity against prosecution) that he had been hired to drive the wagon on the night in question. Feltz claimed that he had chauffeured Van Buskirk, a medical student known as Big Sommers, and another student that he did not know to Lindenwood Cemetery to pick up a body in a sack, and that they had returned to the college with the

33 *Fort Wayne Daily News*, December 27, 1877.

body. (Apparently his fuzzy memory forgot that there actually were two other students, not just one.)

Diehl reported that it had taken a month of investigation to accumulate enough evidence and for the grand jury to convene in order for him to make the arrests. He explained that the overheard discussion between Myers and Clark on the street corner had finally cemented his case; later that same morning, he'd presented his story to Justice of the Peace Ryan whom he sufficiently convinced to issue warrants—on the charge of grave robbing—for the arrests of the drayman Charles Feltz, who was in already in custody; Dr. A.E. Van Buskirk; and two medical students, G.W. Sommers and J.P. ("Big") Sommers. Big was out of town for the Christmas holidays. His arrest would come later. (Though the students' surnames were the same, they were easily told apart by Big's much larger size.)

Those same newspapers that had criticized the plodding Chief Diehl on a daily basis now praised their police chief for outfoxing the interlopers, the glamorous Pinkerton men, who had failed at trying to do his job. With the aplomb of a town hero, Diehl had solved the crime himself. Next, he needed a conviction.

In retrospect, it was odd that Diehl had chosen to approach Justice Ryan for his warrants because the case clearly fell under the jurisdiction of the higher criminal court where such scandalous a crime could be tried and punished to the full extent allowed by law. Given the jurisdictional limitations of the justice of the peace to relatively minor infractions, Lindenwood Cemetery had already declared that its reward offer would not apply to a mere justice of the peace conviction. The judicial choice is even more peculiar considering that Diehl had already admitted his interest in collecting the reward, but perhaps he believed that his circumstantial evidence would be sufficient only to convince the lower court.

The stealing of a body from a grave was specifically and clearly prohibited by statute of Indiana law, but, as it was in most places around the country, body snatching was treated as a relatively minor crime, a misdemeanor, carrying a maximum fine of $1,000.

Even that was well beyond the capabilities of the justice of the peace, who could impose a maximum fine of only $25.

Justice Ryan did accept the case. He set bail for Van Buskirk and G.W. Sommers at $300 each. The men paid their bail and were released with an order to return for their trial at 2:30 p.m. that same afternoon. As anticipated, in exchange for immunity against prosecution, the justice dropped all charges against the wagon driver, Charles Feltz, who had agreed to testify against the doctors.

Van Buskirk and Sommers hired a prominent local attorney, J.Q. Stratton, who happened to be the brother and senior law partner of the prosecuting attorney, Robert Stratton. The choice of the prosecutor also turned out to be controversial for more reasons than the obvious conflict of interest with his brother and firm partner. Another prosecutor, Samuel Hench, had led the prosecution for the grand jury's investigation and was more familiar with the case than his colleagues, and he had wanted to try the case. Moreover, the Lindenwood Cemetery, probably through the voice of Mr. Isaac De Groff Nelson, who was both president of Lindenwood and foreman of the grand jury, had specifically requested that Hench prosecute, but the case was assigned to Robert Stratton instead.

By the time Van Buskirk and G.W. Sommers returned to Justice Ryan's office at the appointed time for their trial, a good-sized crowd had assembled on the street outside. News reports of Chief Diehl's spectacle as he'd paraded his apprehended doctors across Calhoun Street earlier that morning apparently had spread. The attorneys, however, had not been able to gather their witnesses as quickly; it was four o'clock before Justice Ryan began the proceedings, by which time his shabby building was filled with raucous spectators who spilled through the front door out onto the street. Despite the cold December weather, reporters complained of the body heat generated in the jam-packed, stuffy enclosure.

Ryan called the assembly to order, and the defendants rose to hear the charges levied against them.

Both men pleaded not guilty and waived arraignment. They did not need further explanation of the charges being levied against them.

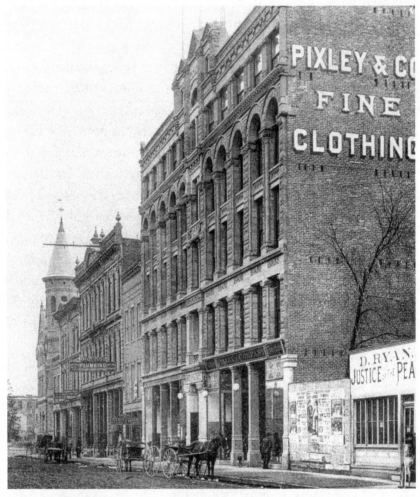

Figure 9. Justice of the Peace Daniel Ryan's ramshackle courtroom, lower right corner. Reproduced with the permission of the Allen County-Fort Wayne Historical Society.

Justice Ryan first called the bereaved Mrs. Charles Wright to the witness stand in his little courtroom. Mary Wright affirmed that she was the widow of Charles Wright who had been buried at Lindenwood Cemetery on November 22. Mrs. Wright believed that her husband had died from abscesses of his head and neck. He had been ill for some time and had been attended by Dr. Gregg and Dr. Woodworth. She described her husband as having been a very tall man, forty-five years of age. She added that he was extremely thin, a condition that had been exacerbated by his prolonged illness. She then described her husband's grave on the gentle slope in the southern area of Lindenwood Cemetery. The defense chose not to cross-examine her.

Next, the venerable Dr. Benjamin Woodworth made his way through the crowd to Ryan's witness-box. Woodworth confirmed the widow's statement that her husband had been afflicted with abscesses of his head and neck, that he was tall, and that his body was so emaciated that it should have been of little value for dissection. He failed to elaborate upon the notion that, in November 1877, the fledgling medical college had been so desperate to provide cadavers to their students that just about any body, regardless of its condition, would no doubt have suited their purposes.

John Doswell, the beleaguered superintendent of Lindenwood Cemetery, testified that his staff was only too aware of the problem of stealing bodies from new graves in the Fort Wayne area. Lindenwood's position, elevated perhaps above many of the local graveyards, offered a modicum of protection, but clearly not enough. Although the grounds already imbued a pastoral sanctity for the living as well as the dead, Doswell's employees had continued to take more practical precautions to protect their graves. He said that, as far as he knew, Lindenwood had been spared the sorts of desecrations that had plagued other smaller graveyards, but the staff understood the temerity and desperation of the local resurrection men. They knew that it was unrealistic to expect that the cemetery was entirely safe. Doswell then described for the court the unique imprint known only to him and the sexton that they impressed upon the soil of each new grave as a mark to assure its security. He added that he had established a routine of personally examining each new grave every morning for "several days" after an interment to ascertain that neither the mark nor the grave had been disturbed.

John Doswell went on to tell the court that he had arisen early on November 23 because he had been worried about Charles Wright's grave. He, too, had seen the suspicious-looking men lurking around during the interment service on November 22. When he made his rounds the next morning, he discovered that the mark had been subtly, but definitely, altered. It could have been from a stray animal rooting in the freshly turned soil, but it appeared more likely that someone had volitionally, if clumsily, rearranged the mark. He confirmed his suspicion when his examination found the coffin opened and vacant. Only the clothes and jewelry of the deceased and the shroud had been left behind.

In their cross-examination, the defense attorney asked Doswell about the $1,000 reward that had been offered by the Lindenwood Cemetery Board of Directors, and suggested that Doswell, in testifying for the prosecution, stood to gain the reward if Van Buskirk and G.W. Sommers were found guilty. Doswell denied the charge in the most vigorous of terms.

Next to the witness stand was Henry Pantlind, one of the stable wagon drivers. Henry liked his beer. He was known to frequent the many beer gardens of Fort Wayne after, if not during, his work at Fletcher and Powers Livery. From the stand, he claimed to have remembered specifically that, on the night of November 22, a party consisting of Van Buskirk and three others had come to the gate at the livery around midnight and had taken a wagon that Charlie Feltz was driving. Van Buskirk and another man sat on the seat, while the others climbed into the back. Pantlind denied that he had any personal acquaintance with Van Buskirk, and he could not remember what the accused had been wearing on the night of November 22. He thought that Sommers could have been in the party. (*Note:* He did not specify whether he thought that "Sommers" referred to G.W, the pharmacist as well as medical student, or to Big Sommers, a preceptor-trained doctor who was now a medical student hoping for an MD degree—or that both had been there.) Pantlind also confirmed that he was not the one who had been asked to drive the wagon; only Charles Feltz had. The defense suggested that Pantlind could be induced to say about anything, as long as it was over a pint.

The manager of Fletcher and Powers, Mr. M.E. Woodward, confirmed the essence of his employee's remarks, reporting at first that Van Buskirk had come to the livery about eight o'clock in the evening of November 22 to arrange a wagon and driver for later that night, around midnight. He had told them that Charles Feltz was working that night and would be their hack driver. Woodward then stated that he went home shortly thereafter and did not see Dr. Van Buskirk again. However, he reported that the doctor had paid him $3 for the wagon and driver for about an hour and a half's service, and that the books would show the payment. On cross-examination, however, Woodward wavered with second thoughts. He admitted that he did not know Van Buskirk well enough to recognize him in the dark, and that he really was not sure who had hired the wagon; he only assumed that it was Van Buskirk and that, in the dark, the man had resembled the doctor. But Woodward then admitted that it could have been someone else with whom he had contracted for the midnight wagon, and that perhaps the doctor had only been there paying the college's bill for general livery services. The prosecutor redirected his witness to press his strong belief that it was, in fact, Van Buskirk who had paid for the wagon, but the seeds of doubt had already sprouted.

Next came the hack driver, Charles Feltz, who had run a saloon in a small neighboring village before he'd taken the job as wagon driver at Fletcher and Powers a few months before. He had drawn the 10:00 a.m. to midnight shift. Although it was his first autumn as a hack driver in Fort Wayne, Feltz seemed to know Van Buskirk, himself a relative newcomer to the city. With his newly granted immunity, Charles Feltz had become the prosecution's star witness. He testified that he had been ordered by Mr. Woodward to have the wagon ready at midnight to drive the men, as directed by the doctor, who presumably was A.E. Van Buskirk. Feltz described how he had his rig hitched up and ready to go by the time his customers, Van Buskirk, G.W. Sommers, and two others arrived at the livery. As the doctor directed, he drove west on Main Street over the St. Mary's Bridge, then crossed the old canal into Lindenwood Cemetery. The doctor then gave him specific instructions to drive the wagon west and then to the southeast corner of the Lindenwood grounds. Feltz stated that when they stopped, the doctor ordered him to turn the wagon around so as to be ready to leave as quickly as possible. Then, Feltz (*incorrectly*) claimed that Van Buskirk whistled, and two men came out of the woods, carrying a long sack that appeared to contain a body. The men pitched their load into the back of the wagon. Sommers climbed on the seat next to the driver while Van Buskirk and a "heavy set" man got onto the bed of the wagon with their package. (*Again, this was incorrect, for A.E. climbed onto the front seat, not into the back.*) The doctor then instructed Feltz to drive to the medical college on the corner of Washington and Broadway, so he steered the wagon back up Main Street and turned right onto Broadway for the three blocks south to Washington. Feltz knew that the school was on the upper floors of the Remmel Building over Wright's Drug Store. Dr. Van Buskirk threw the bulky bundle over his shoulder (*also incorrect*) and entered the building through a side door on Broadway Street. Feltz reasserted that the parcel appeared to hold the body of a human being, but, naturally, he did not look inside. After discharging his passengers, he returned directly to the barn and arrived there around 2:30 a.m., a bit later than he had expected, but he was glad to be done with it.

Though his testimony was laden with incorrect details, the overall content seemed believable.

Through the careful orchestration of the prosecuting attorney, Feltz then described the profound shock he had experienced the following morning when he learned that the authorities had discovered the theft of a body from Lindenwood Cemetery during the night. Announcement of the $1,000 reward only intensified his anxiety. He claimed that he sought out Van Buskirk twice to talk to him about what could be done. Although Feltz denied that he had received anything for his silence, he also said he'd been told that he would "want for nothing." He went on to explain that he and the doctor had discussed whether Feltz should leave town but finally agreed that he should remain in Fort Wayne. He declared that Van Buskirk and Sommers had told him not to "give them away." On the other hand, Feltz also specifically stated that they had not told him to remain silent on the matter, leaving the court unclear about what had actually transpired between the hack driver and the doctors.

Defense attorney Stratton cross-examined Feltz, who then claimed that before his customers arrived, he had no idea where they would be going that night, but he added that Woodward had given him extra pay for what the manager had thought would be an extra difficult night's work. Feltz avowed that it was the only job of that sort that he had ever performed, but, later, he admitted that he went on midnight sojourns to the local graveyards quite often. He said that he had seen Van Buskirk previously, presumably at the livery, before the Wright case, but that he did not know him personally. He stated that after the reward was offered, he went to Van Buskirk because he didn't want to get into trouble and he wanted to know what should be done. The drayman denied asking for any money or attempting to blackmail anyone. Further, he had not received any money and he did not expect to receive any of Lindenwood's $1,000 reward. Fletcher and Powers paid him $1 for a day's work, and that was good enough for him. He claimed that he had finally gone to Chief Diehl because the police seemed to have learned about it anyway, and that he wanted to get out of the scrape as best as he could.

The final witness that Thursday was the first of the medical students, Herschel Myers, whose father, Professor W.H. Myers, had been having difficulty with the college, the hospital, and the other doctors. It was the senior Myers who, with his colleague Professor Clark, allegedly had tipped off Chief Diehl about Van Buskirk. Herschel testified that on the night of November 23, the day following Wright's resurrection, there were several cadavers on the tables, but that the only fresh one was that of a tall, thin male with large abscesses on the side of his neck and a fractured skull. He stated that had never seen Wright in life or death, and that he had no idea about the identity of the cadaver that was lying on the table. He declared that the demonstrator of anatomy, Dr. Van Buskirk, was there that night, as were G.W. Sommers and other students who were performing the dissection. Young Myers also stated that, on Sunday, November 25, 1877, the day after the reward was offered, he observed a heated discussion in the street in front of his house between his father and Drs. Clark and Van Buskirk and a medical student named Moffat. Herschel Myers claimed that he could hear them arguing about the appropriate disposition of Wright's body. He said he heard Van Buskirk suggest that the head should be removed to prevent identification of the corpse. Furthermore, the following day, Myers observed the cadaver lying on one of the dissection tables without its head, and he noted that later the body had been removed as well.

At that point, the exhausted Squire Daniel Ryan suspended further proceedings until nine o'clock the following morning, Friday, December 28.

Soon after dawn, curious onlookers again began to gather on Berry Street in front of Justice Ryan's modest chambers. By nine o'clock, the room was packed with reporters and spectators who were lusting for sordid details. Squire Ryan resumed his trial with the prosecution recalling the medical student, Herschel Myers.

Myers was asked to repeat his testimony about the activities in the dissection room on the night of the November 23 and the description of the emaciated "stiff" on one of the tables. The witness reaffirmed that he thought the skull was fractured, but that the injury was not a recent one. He claimed that he was in the dissection room quite frequently and was sure that that particular body had not been there before.

Under J.Q. Stratton's cross-examination for the defense, however, the student wasn't quite so sure of himself or of what he had really seen. Young Myers retreated from the firm stance he had assumed before the prosecutor. He declared that he was only a medical student, not a graduate physician. Perhaps he had over-interpreted what he had seen. As the questions continued, his recollection of the conversation between his father and the other doctors shifted from his previously definitive recitation of their words to only a "general conversation." He now admitted that, in fact, Wright's name had never been mentioned. Caught in an obvious inconsistency, young Herschel Myers flushed and grew impatient with Stratton's cross-examination. Angrily, he asserted that he had already answered those questions before the grand jury earlier in the month. Stratton pressed him; he implied that the flustered student might be trying to get the $1,000 reward, but young Myers held his ground. He admitted that he had been pumped hard by Chief Diehl and by the prosecutors, but he vigorously denied that he had been offered any reward by them or by anyone else.

In the midst of impugning what seemed to be crucial testimony of a damning witness, the defense abruptly cooled the intensity of his questions, as if he had lost interest in what young Myers had to say. The student's comments about his previous testimony before the grand jury apparently had tweaked the defense attorney's memory, as if Stratton suddenly recalled something from the grand jury investigation that had taken place right after the body snatching had been discovered. He quickly wound down his interrogation of the student, dismissed him, and recalled the wagon driver, Charles Feltz.

The grand jury had interviewed everyone who could possibly have been involved, including cemetery and livery people, the doctors, and the students—many of whom were now testifying before Justice Ryan. The grand jury had been rather ineffectual. However, when Stratton was questioning young Myers, he remembered that the hack driver, Charles Feltz, had, at that time, avowed no knowledge of the affair, of the events that he had described so vividly in the courtroom the day before. When Stratton got him back on the stand, he challenged the wagon driver about his blatant prevarication.

Obviously shaken by the revelation, Charles Feltz then admitted that he had lied to the grand jury when he'd stated he had never hauled a package from Lindenwood Cemetery, but he denied Stratton's assertion that he had told the grand jury he knew nothing of the matter. Further, he claimed that he had not seen Van Buskirk on the night of November 22, but at that point Feltz seemed desperate to restore his credibility and avoid a perjury charge. Feltz now admitted that he did know some of the doctors—Myers, Clark, and Woodworth—but he contended he had never hauled bodies for them. He claimed that Van Buskirk's name was not even mentioned in his testimony before the grand jury because he was never asked about Van Buskirk. (*That, in fact, was true.*) As the defense attorney homed in, the feckless wagon driver's frustration mounted. His testimony grew more confused and contradictory; he became dithering. Justice Ryan dismissed him and called for a recess. The justice needed lunch.

At two o clock in the afternoon, Squire Ryan again faced a packed courtroom room that collectively sensed an imminent climax. Prosecutor Robert Stratton called Professor Harold A. Clark, but, curiously, the reclusive anatomist was nowhere to be found. No one present could account for his absence nor could anyone recall having seen him in the few days before the trial.

Clark's name had been mentioned frequently during the course of the trial because he was the professor of anatomy, Van Buskirk's supervisor, and he was a close friend and confidant of Professor Myers. Despite his obvious culpability as head of the anatomy program, Clark had managed to skulk in Professor Myers's ample shadow while transferring responsibility to his young subordinate. In addition, the overheard conversation between Myers and Clark had provided Chief Diehl with the crucial information that underpinned his arrest of Van Buskirk and G.W. Sommers. The professor's testimony would have been vital, but the reclusive doctor had disappeared. To the prosecution's further embarrassment, the senior Myers also had vanished, apparently having gone on vacation for the Christmas holidays.

In the absence of Clark and Myers, the prosecution lumbered on by calling the various medical students who might have had either a role in the affair or at least some knowledge of the events of November 23 when Wright's body was alleged to have been dissected. Then, Robert Stratton made a peculiar choice by calling R.P. Morris, a student, to attest that, for certain, Dr. A.E. Van Buskirk was demonstrator of anatomy and, as such, was in charge of the dissection room. However, Morris testified that he was not in the dissecting rooms on November 23, nor did he know anything about a body with abscesses on its head. It is not clear why the prosecution should have selected this particular student for he seemed to add nothing to their argument.

Perhaps in resignation, Stratton rested the prosecution's case. Ryan appeared puzzled; he recessed the trial for the day. The defense would have their opportunity to call their witnesses the following morning.

On Saturday, J.Q. Stratton, the defense attorney, recalled the much-venerated Dr. Benjamin Woodworth who had been one of Charles Wright's physicians. He explained that although Wright's head and neck were covered with abscesses, the sores may not have been visible to casual observation but were obviously "perceptible" to the touch. Woodworth doubted that the abscesses had eroded into the skull; the old doctor could not account for the report by some of the students that the skull was fractured. Responding to the prosecution's cross-examination, Dr. Woodworth claimed he was not aware of any head trauma in Wright's case. Perhaps the fracture had occurred posthumously, during the rough extraction from the coffin with resurrectionist's bar, or perhaps they had fabricated the entire story. After all, by then there was no prospect to confirm or deny a skull fracture for the head had long been buried among the roots of a nearby tree.

The defense next called Samuel Hench who was the other prosecuting attorney for the county but who had not been assigned to prosecute Squire Ryan's trial. Because grand jury investigations did not become part of the public record and no reporters had been present during the proceedings, Hench was called as the most reliable witness to describe what had been said. His recollections became crucial for both sides.

Samuel Hench confirmed that he had questioned Charles Feltz before the grand jury in early December. In that setting, Feltz had sworn he did not know anything about the Wright affair; he also had denied that he had hauled any package from Lindenwood Cemetery, or from the neighborhood, or even from that direction. According to Hench, Feltz had stated in the strongest of terms that he had never visited the cemetery at night.

The prosecutors then cross-examined their colleague from the district attorney's office, and they began to probe what must have been their own recollections of idle chat around the office. Prosecutor Stratton asked Hench if it wasn't common knowledge that he disliked Police Chief Hugh Diehl. Stratton pressed his contention that perhaps Hench was out to harm the police chief by discrediting how he'd handled the body-snatching case.

Vigorously denying the charge, Hench acknowledged that he had opposed Diehl politically but not personally. He admitted that he had, in the past, criticized the ways in which Diehl had handled some cases. As if to confound the proceedings further, Hench then explained that, although he had represented the district attorney's office with the grand jury, he had not been asked prosecute the case when it came to trial. Further, he revealed that the Lindenwood officials had actually requested that he prosecute, but that the case had gone to Stratton instead.

As for Lindenwood Cemetery, Hench also reported that the president of its board of directors, I.D.G. Nelson, who also had been the foreman of the grand jury, had actually expressed concern that the case would not be handled properly if Hench were not prosecuting or if it were tried in the lowly court of the Justice of the Peace. Nelson knew that in that court, even if the perpetrators were found guilty, they could receive, at most, only a nominal fine. At that point, the cemetery president had declared that they would not pay a reward for a mere justice of the peace conviction, that they would only pay the $1,000 reward if the case were tried in the circuit court. According to Hench, despite those backroom machinations, Chief Diehl brought his case to the justice of the peace and Robert Stratton, not Samuel Hench, had been assigned to prosecute.

A series of medical students, each having some information about the nights of November 22 and 23, were then called. First up was R.F. Lipes, a student who was personally close to the defendants. Lipes testified that he had been with G.W. Sommers the night of November 22. Lipes affirmed that, naturally, he knew both Van Buskirk and Sommers well, the former being his professor, the latter, his fellow student. Next up, another student, S.D. Sledd, confirmed that G.W. Sommers, indeed, had been in his room at 236 South Broadway studying from 8:00 p.m. to 1:00 a.m. during the night of the resurrection.

It was then established that there were two medical students named Sommers. The student called "Big" Sommers was a practicing physician in Fort Wayne, licensed on the basis of a preceptorship;

he had enrolled in the medical college to obtain his MD degree.[34] But Big Sommers was vacationing out of the city and had not yet been contacted. The other Sommers student, G. William Sommers, had been a practicing pharmacist in Fort Wayne for some eight years before he matriculated at the local college of medicine, and he was the one who now stood accused in the Wright case. He was called next.

G. William Sommers avowed that, as stated by Sledd, he had been in Sledd's room on the night of November 22. He denied he had ever been to Fletcher and Powers's stable, and he stated that he knew nothing of the Wright affair; he had never stolen a body and had never visited Lindenwood at night. It would have been untenable to have stated that he had never been to Lindenwood at all, for nearly everyone went there on occasion to pay their respects or just to stroll and picnic on Sunday afternoons. Sommers emphasized that he had not been to Lindenwood in any capacity for over a year. He did, however, go on to admit that on November 23 he had seen a cadaver with a tumor on the neck in the dissecting laboratory—thus conforming to the previous description of Wright's body. He said he had seen no abscesses on the head, but he had only seen the body from across the room. Asserting that his classmate Herschel Myers had lied about the events of November 23, Sommers contended that, in fact, it had been Herschel who had been dissecting the tall, emaciated corpse. The newspaper reporter who recorded G. William Sommers's testimony added that, in contrast to many of the other witnesses, Sommers gave his in such a frank, open, and credible manner, that he made a very favorable impression on the court and jury.

Dr. Morrison, another practicing physician and medical student, testified that he had intended to dissect at seven o'clock

---

34 Many physicians had obtained their training by apprenticing to another physician before getting a medical license and practicing on their own. By 1877, it had become advantageous to hold a doctor of medicine degree and, as A.E. Van Buskirk had done a few years earlier, many licensed physicians entered medical colleges as students.

in the evening of Friday, November 23, but that when he arrived he had found the anatomical laboratories locked, barring his entry. In cross-examination, he added that the rooms may have been unlocked later, after he left, but he thought not. He noted that he had run into some other students who were distraught over the news of Wright's exhumation. They had been conducting their own investigation into each other's whereabouts on the night of November 22. At least six of them knew exactly what had happened because they were directly involved, either by having been in the wagon or dissecting in the laboratory.

Finally, the defense called the accused, Demonstrator of Anatomy A.E. Van Buskirk, who ascended to the stand to testify on his own behalf. The *Sentinel* reporter observed that Van Buskirk appeared disheveled and rather confused. In contrast to Sommers, A.E.'s delivery was so uncertain and vacillating that he left a most unfavorable impression on everyone present from the justice to the fidgety crowd of onlookers. He denied visiting either Fletcher and Powers Livery or Lindenwood Cemetery. He vociferously denied stealing Wright's body. He testified that he was at the college on the night of November 22, but that he had gone home around 10:00 p.m. On cross-examination, he reasserted his denials without contributing any new information in his defense. He could not recall reserving or paying for any rig. Van Buskirk further emphasized that if he had hired a wagon at so late an hour, he certainly would have remembered it. He admitted that he might have done business with Fletcher and Powers at some point in time because, like most people, he was in occasional need of appropriate livery, but he could not recall any particular instance. He denied that he had any acquaintance with either M.E. Woodward, the manager at the stable, or H. Pantlind, the beer-drinking employee who had testified for the prosecution.

Curiously, Van Buskirk simply refused to comment on the question of whether or not he had tried to conceal Wright's body or had played a role in taking off the head. The demonstrator observed that he oversaw the dissection of every cadaver, but he explained that he did not make a habit of recalling the specific features of any individual. He claimed that he had not known Charles Wright in life and did not recall dissecting his particular body. He admitted, of course, that he knew the students Moffat and Herschel Myers as well as the professors Clark and Myers.

Compounding the confusion, there were actually three different Dr. Myers involved in the case: Professor W.H. Myers and Dr. I.N. Myers were brothers and fellow physicians; Herschel Myers was the medical student who was Professor Myers's son. Further, another Myers relative was a building contractor; one of the conclaves to plan the doctors' response to the discovery of the resurrection had transpired at his house.

In contradiction to Herschel Myers's testimony about the conversation he had overheard in the street in front of his father's house, Van Buskirk testified that he had no recollection of any such street meeting. He did not remember any conversation about the concealment of Wright's body. He did acknowledge that he was responsible for furnishing subjects for dissection to the college of medicine and that he was responsible for the dissections themselves. He confirmed that he usually examined each subject himself and that, undoubtedly, he saw them all at some stage during their dissection. He admitted that at some time during the winter he had seen a male subject on the table with a tumor on its neck and that he had noted that the skull had been fractured. Although he couldn't recall exactly when that had been, he agreed with previous testimony that it was probably during November. In cross-examination, he repeated his denials already made, but finally reluctantly divulged that he had, on occasion, met the Fletcher and Powers drayman, Charles Feltz.

At that point, Squire Ryan expressed the need to hear from Professor W.H. Myers. He adjourned the court until nine o'clock Sunday morning with the hope that Myers could be located. But in the morning, Prosecutor Stratton, obviously embarrassed by the lapse, grudgingly acknowledged that he could not locate either Dr. W.H. Myers, the bombastic surgeon who seemed to have tipped off Captain Diehl, or Myers's ephemeral partner, Harold A. Clark. Both men had "mysteriously" disappeared. Without being able to produce further testimony, the prosecutor said he felt they had sufficient evidence to make their case. Justice Ryan then allowed each side one hour for concluding arguments, after which he adjourned at three o'clock with the promise that he would take the matter under advisement and render a decision at nine o'clock on Monday morning.

In the muted light of winter's dawn, plumes of icy breath drifted through the crisp morning air as reporters and spectators gathered on Berry Street, outside Justice Ryan's court. Some fortified themselves against the cold next door in the Aveline's café, its windows still draped with limp holiday garlands that spewed dried needles on the sill below. At a quarter to nine, the doors opened to admit as many spectators as the cramped space would hold. Squire Ryan made his way to the bench at the nine o'clock hour. The crowd was silent as he called for the defendants to stand before him; then he rose before the anxious crowd. He cleared his throat to address his hushed courtroom. If the spectators had expected a climactic scenario, an audible exhalation of disappointment must have exuded over the little room, for Ryan announced simply that the case against the anatomist, Dr. A.E. Van Buskirk, was beyond his ken. He went on to state in the strongest of terms that, while he had no doubt about Van Buskirk's guilt, it was beyond the power of a justice of the peace to assess an adequate punishment for such a heinous crime. Therefore, he had requested that the prosecution enter a *nolle prosequi* plea, a decision not to prosecute. He then "certified the case up to criminal court."[35]

---

35 *Nolle Prosequi* is derived from the Latin term that means the court is not willing to prosecute, in this case ostensibly because they were unable to produce key witnesses, but perhaps because Justice Ryan knew he was out of his depth. It does call for the case to be retried as it was in the criminal court.

In the meantime, Squire Ryan found the pharmacist/student G.W. (William) Sommers innocent of all charges, and he was dismissed. Van Buskirk was then again charged, and again released on $300 bail, which was covered by his colleagues. His case was remanded to the criminal court for another grand jury investigation and probably another trial.

CHAPTER 13

Tried Again

HANKS TO THE GENEROSITY of his faculty colleague, Dr. T.J. Dills and two of his students, Lipes and Moffat, who guaranteed his $300 bond, A.E. Van Buskirk celebrated New Year's Day, 1878, with his wife, Mary Jane, in relative freedom. It was a freedom tempered by the fact that another grand jury investigation loomed ahead, from which an indictment seemed inevitable. That time, A.E.'s trial would be held in criminal court under Judge Borden. Between A.E.'s contradictory testimony, the obvious dissembling of young Herschel Myers, the hack driver Charles Feltz, and some of the other students, all had proved too much for Justice of the Peace Ryan. Their prevarications also led the *Fort Wayne Daily News* of Saturday, December 29 to question in its headline: "Who's a Liar?" Only the accused pharmacist, G. William Sommers, had left an impression of veracity that had earned him a prompt acquittal.

And though neither the senior W.H. Myers, erstwhile professor of surgery, distinguished medical college founder, and faculty combatant, nor his ephemeral colleague Harold Clark, could be found to testify in Van Buskirk's first trial, but both suddenly surfaced at its conclusion.

With the type of careful orchestration for which he was well known, Professor W.H. Myers reappeared to give an interview to a reporter for the *Fort Wayne Sentinel*. In that interview, Myers contended unequivocally that he personally had had no connection with the stealing of Wright's body, but that he knew all about the case, and he knew for certain that Van Buskirk was guilty. He didn't know anything about Sommers. He maintained that he had advised Van Buskirk, as a friend, to plead guilty as the best way to conclude the matter as quickly and as painlessly as possible. Myers then told the reporter that his testimony would reveal the whole matter when Van Buskirk came to trial in criminal court. "I shall expose the entire affair from beginning to end."

Clark, on the other hand, from his lair in the background, wrote a series of bombastic letters to the local newspapers castigating his former colleague, Van Buskirk, but Clark was actually never seen again in the city of Fort Wayne.

Another reporter interviewed an adamantly anonymous doctor at the medical college who claimed to know about Wright's body. He stated that as soon as the reward had been posted, three doctors had proceeded to the dissection rooms and locked themselves in. They then removed Wright's head, wrapped it in an old sack, and burned it in the furnace. They stripped all the flesh, which was similarly combusted. The anonymous doctor then said that the three doctors boiled the body "to fluid" and retained the skeleton as a specimen for the college.

Dr. Van Buskirk had had his troubles with both Professor Myers and Professor Clark from his first days at the Medical College of Fort Wayne. On August 13, 1877, before he had even taught his first class, A.E. had been appointed secretary of the faculty—a position that had saddled the newcomer with daunting administrative responsibilities for which he was ill prepared. Professors Myers and Clark subsequently blamed A.E. for their difficulties with the other members of the faculty and with St. Joseph Hospital. (Myers later testified that, after the snafus over Whitey Dan, as long as Myers was a member of the hospital medical staff, Van Buskirk would allow no medical college patients to be admitted to the hospital.)

Although Van Buskirk was disgusted with Clark, perhaps more for what he saw as Clark's duplicitous backing of Myers than for any specific grievances, he blamed Myers both for his own troubles and those of the medical college. According to Van Buskirk, Myers and Clark had antagonized their colleagues when they'd failed to back Dr. Dills and Buchman in their refusal to provide expert testimony in the earlier Hamilton case without compensation. Van Buskirk felt that, now, having been unable to manipulate the faculty to their own liking, Myers and Clark were trying to destroy the young college and start a new one of their own. (Remarkably, the roots of his prescience had sprung from a well that went deeper than just his own personal bitterness.)

On Friday, January 11, 1878, the grand jury indicted A.E. Van Buskirk and the medical student J.P. "Big" Sommers—the "other" Sommers—for stealing the body of Charles Wright. The defendants posted $1,000 bail each. The struggling young Dr. Van Buskirk had already been obliged to turn to his colleague and even to his students to cover his $300 bail obligation. Again, Dr. T.J. Dills and the two students, Lipes and Moffat, provided surety for A.E. Although Big Sommers had been out of town and had missed the entire proceedings of the justice of the peace, he had been among those listed on Squire Ryan's original arrest warrant. Van Buskirk and Big Sommers were to be tried separately, Van Buskirk first, beginning on Monday, January 21.

The taint of scandal ran broad and deep throughout the struggling medical college. As the students worried about their fate, they debated what they perceived to be the roots of the schism that now divided their faculty. They were conflicted among themselves about who was really to blame and what course of action they should take. The students who had complained in early November about the shortage of cadavers to the school's board of directors had undoubtedly contributed to the problem. But now, the very existence of their school was in jeopardy.

At first, most of the students had sided with Dr. Van Buskirk. They prepared and signed a petition recommending that Myers and Clark be expelled from the faculty as the best course of action to restore order to the school. Two of A.E.'s most ardent supporters, Lipes and Moffat, had gone so far as to contribute their own money to cover his bail, not once, but twice. Then, a small faction of students who recalled Professor Myers's excellent teaching and his dedication to the school spoke out on behalf of the professor of surgery and of his colleague, Professor Clark. Those students went so far as to draft a second petition to be delivered to Professors Myers and Clark urging them not to resign. By then, however, the matter had exploded beyond the purview of medical students.

If Myers and Clark had sought the school's demise, their wishes were near fulfillment. In addition to the indictments of Van Buskirk and Big Sommers, the grand jury issued a separate charge against the medical college itself, declaring it to be a public nuisance. On January 11, 1878, the *Fort Wayne Daily News* questioned whether or not the school could survive as scandal piled upon scandal.

On Monday, January 21, spectators who had been following the Wright case crammed into a new courtroom, the criminal court in the Allen County Courthouse, (*see Fig. 10*), across the street from Justice of the Peace Ryan's modest quarters. Despite the more suitable location, the reporters still complained about the stuffy body heat that permeated the crowded room.

On Monday and Tuesday, the testimony emanated from the same parade of witnesses who had marched to and from Justice Ryan's stand. They reiterated the same tales they'd already told. Charles Feltz proclaimed his innocence with the same inconsistent prevarications; the doctors and local druggists spoke for and against the demonstrator. Medical students did likewise.

Dr. Benjamin Woodworth provided a modicum of entertainment when he expressed his resentment about questioning the validity of his diagnosis. In the absence of specific therapy for

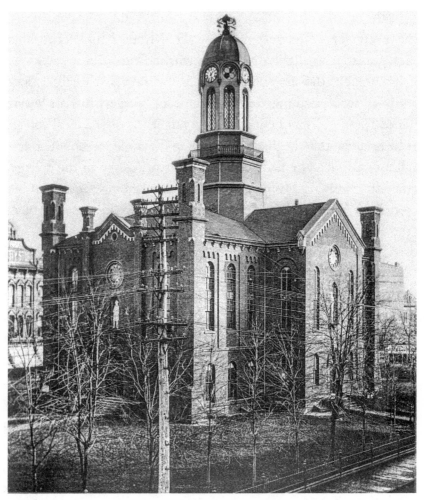

Figure 10. Allen County Courthouse as it appeared in 1878. Reproduced with the permission of the Allen County-Fort Wayne Historical Society.

most disorders, the public perception of the doctor's ability to diagnose and prognosticate accurately constituted the foundation of a successful medical practice. Venerated as he was, perhaps old Dr. Woodworth could not permit any doubt to be reflected upon his current capability. As he described the nature of Wright's malaria and scrofula, he dismissed the absurdity of requesting a consultation for so mundane a situation. Similar cases were seen every day. For the same reason, he had not ordered an autopsy.

The prosecution's key witness on Wednesday proved to be Professor of Surgery William H. Myers, MD, A.E.'s chief antagonist, who alighted upon the witness stand like a hawk on a high branch. The surgeon recounted his impressive qualifications, noting that he had practiced medicine and surgery in Fort Wayne since 1866, and that he lectured on surgery at the medical college. He recalled that he had known Van Buskirk for about a year, although it actually had been at least two. As one of the college's founding fathers, Myers would have been among those who had recruited A.E. Van Buskirk well before the Aveline meeting when the board of directors formally completed their proposal.

As the imposing surgeon prepared to speak, a palpable lull descended over the courtroom like a restless congregation settling in for a lengthy sermon. Myers knew how to work an audience and which of his words would carry the most weight. Respected as a surgeon by everyone in the room, he was also feared by many for the influence his family wielded in the city. His challenge was to castigate his colleague sufficiently to extract a modicum of revenge, while constructing a shield around himself without entirely undermining the credibility of the college that he had worked so hard to assemble.

The prosecutor began his questions, but the intimidating Myers quickly grabbed the floor for himself. He testified that Van Buskirk served as demonstrator of anatomy, that he lectured on surgical anatomy, and that he was responsible for the dissection room. Indeed, Dr. Van Buskirk was in charge of furnishing anatomical subjects for the students' dissection. Myers confirmed that the demonstrator had been the one who was obtaining the bodies during the previous November.

He further claimed to have seen Van Buskirk one or two nights after the Wright burial and that he, Myers, was actually with him in the dissecting room. He added that he could not remember any specific bodies on the tables at that particular time. However, he clearly remembered the day that the Lindenwood Cemetery discovered the theft of Wright's body, Friday, November 23. Myers reported that he had been alarmed by the discovery and that, upon hearing the news, he immediately summoned Van Buskirk to his chambers and had emphasized the necessity of arranging prompt disposition of the body to protect the institution. Myers claimed to have offered suggestions to Van Buskirk, but he said the anatomist was not receptive to his ideas. Instead, Van Buskirk allegedly told him that the police already had unsuccessfully attempted to enter the college and that if they had breached the dissecting chamber's door, which had been guarded by one of the students, they would have found the body of Charles Wright.

Myers went on to claim that later the same day, Van Buskirk and the medical student Moffat came to him "much excited." They complained that the police had surrounded the medical college building, and that they could not enter. Myers described how he then went with the demonstrator to the college but that, by the time they had arrived, the police had left. Myers and Van Buskirk entered the dissection laboratory where the demonstrator showed him the body lying headless upon one of the tables. Myers testified that Van Buskirk had told him that he had removed the head to prevent identification of the corpse. The defendant paled and turned to his attorney who calmed the doctor with a barely perceptible nod of his head. The surgeon had paused for a breath as if to let the impact of his oratory inculcate itself into the minds of the spectators and jurors.

The prosecutor urged Myers to continue. The surgeon testified that both he and Dr. Van Buskirk then left the college, but that he arranged for Van Buskirk to meet him at the home of his cousin, William Myers, the contractor, later that evening, in order to discuss an appropriate course of action. Dr. Myers stated that he had suggested meeting at the cousin's home because it was in a convenient and unobtrusive location, but that the building contractor was not present when they were there. Myers claimed that while in his cousin's home, he had urged the young demonstrator to admit his guilt, claiming that if he did, he would only be assessed a nominal fee. He then could get on with his own life, and it would cause the least amount of damage to the school. But Myers said Van Buskirk refused to take the blame because by then he was worried that the town uproar would demand more than a hand slap and assessment of a nominal fee. Myers said that A.E. then left to consult with Dr. Hiram Van Sweringen, another faculty member who happened to be Professor Myers's brother-in-law.

The prosecutor, Robert Stratton, concluded his examination of the witness and yielded to his brother, attorney for the defense.

J.Q. Stratton glanced at the nervous A.E. who sat slightly slumped to one side. Then J.Q. rose from his chair and strode directly to the witness-box, pausing to glower over the witness as if to let the daunting surgeon know that he, unlike many of those present, would not be intimidated by a grumpy physician. He began his cross-examination by probing the doctor's relationship with Dr. Van Buskirk, especially in light of the recent rancorous exchange of letters published in the local newspapers between Van Buskirk and Myers's compatriot, Harold A. Clark. In the printed correspondence, the beleaguered demonstrator had referred to Myers as an "uncaged anthropoid ape." Myers, at first, asserted that he had no "unfriendly" feelings toward the defendant; he was simply trying to recount the events as they had occurred. He denied that he had had any difficulty with the faculty until the lawyer reminded him that he had found it necessary to take the extreme measure of applying for a restraining order against the college to prevent them from expelling him from their faculty. As J.Q. Stratton dug deeper, Myers admitted he was furious with Van Buskirk when the anatomist had penned antagonistic articles about him both in the local papers and in a St. Louis medical journal. He claimed he did not mind that A.E. had filed an affidavit to prevent any patients of the college being admitted to the hospital while Myers remained a member of its medical staff. Myers explained that he had simply taken the hospital matter to court and had obtained a restraining order to prevent St. Joseph Hospital from expelling him. He added that his only desire was to be able to care for his own patients.

Myers went on to testify that when he and Van Buskirk had returned later to the dissecting rooms, they found the body lying in parts upon the table, with some portions strewn on the floor underneath. He then claimed that he had actually helped Van Buskirk rapidly complete the dissection and dispose of the flesh, and it all had required approximately two hours. He again explained how Van Buskirk had apparently had the head buried under a tree, near the organ factory, but he noted that later the skull had reappeared in the college as a "pathological specimen" for their anatomical museum.

J.Q. then inquired about Myers's colleague, the elusive Professor Clark, who again had vanished. For a few days after the first trial, Clark apparently had returned to Fort Wayne, perhaps to get his affairs in order. Though he and Van Buskirk had exchanged those caustic, accusatory letters in the newspapers, Clark was not actually seen in person then, or ever again. Anxious to distance himself from his evanescent colleague, Myers claimed he had no idea what had happened to Clark. He denied most vigorously that Clark, himself, or his brother, I.N. Myers, had anything to do with the snatch of Wright's body. He noted that Clark and I.N. Myers "were on the outs."

As professor of anatomy, Harold A. Clark had been ultimately responsible for the dissecting rooms at the medical college, but it had been well established that he had delegated all of the anatomy department's daily operations to Dr. Van Buskirk. As the demonstrator's superior, Clark knew that he was accountable for what took place there, but he didn't want any part of the actual dissection. It was the two of them, Van Buskirk and Clark together, who had borne the brunt of the faculty criticism for not providing enough cadavers to the medical students. When it became clear that the case would not rest until it reached its natural conclusion, Professor Clark simply had left town, bolting for the West, never to return.

The biographer of nineteenth-century Ohioan physicians, Otto Juettner, described Harold Clark as a gifted, but "ill-balanced," impulsive man.[36] At the height of the Civil War, the Union Army had discharged him early because of "illness." He had taken a job as doctor to the Ohio State Prison before becoming professor of chemistry in Cincinnati, but resigned after three years to become professor of anatomy in Fort Wayne. After his precipitate departure for the West, he turned up in Eureka, Kansas, where he clerked in a drug store, then started a newspaper and lost everything he had. Finally, Clark moved to a small neighboring town of Severy, Kansas, where he started a new practice of medicine, but he died a short time later in 1882.

In contrast to Clark, Professor Myers had no compunction about confronting his antagonists, but the bombastic surgeon faced a difficult dilemma. He wished to distance himself as far as possible from the Wright mess but, at the same time, he did not want to relinquish his control of the medical college. In fairness, Myers was unquestionably dedicated to teaching surgery and was perhaps the most vocal advocate in the city for human dissection as the foundation of good surgery. Never shrinking from a difficult problem, Professor Myers unabashedly and repeatedly admitted his own expertise in the practice of body snatching. He felt that the process of taking bodies from their new graves was a necessary, if distasteful, skill required for teaching medicine and surgery. On more than one occasion, he'd spoken—not without a tinge of

---

36 Otto Juettner, MD, *Daniel Drake and his Followers* (Cincinnati: Harvey Publishing Company, 1909), 283.

pride—about his exploits in the exhumation of the body of a Mrs. Schiner from the graveyard in Van Wert, Ohio, which was only a few miles east of Fort Wayne. He'd shown no compunction about that extraordinary admission, and, even as the Wright furor swirled through the college of medicine, he brazenly had attempted to divert the decomposing body of the tramp Whitey Dan from his autopsy table in St. Joseph Hospital to the medical college for his students' ministrations. He was still annoyed that his efforts had been blocked by Bishop Dwenger and the hospital.

Back in the courtroom, J.Q. Stratton began to explore the issue of Professor Myers's credibility. Nearly everyone in town knew the surgeon; almost no one was neutral in their feelings about Myers—his family was a powerful lot in Fort Wayne. As a graduate of the prestigious Jefferson Medical College in Philadelphia, Dr. Myers was commonly recognized as Fort Wayne's foremost surgeon, and descriptions of his sometimes "heroic" operations often found their way into columns of the local newspapers. He also was the respected surgeon to the Pennsylvania Railroad. On the other hand, the ill-tempered Dr. Myers sparked controversy wherever he went over what often seemed to be relatively minor affronts. He had generated more than a few enemies among his colleagues in medicine and in the community at large, frequently finding himself in court over various suits and insults.

Without hesitation, defense attorney J.Q. next probed the surgeon's questionable discharge from the Army during the Civil War. After passage of barely a decade since Appomattox, the War of the Republic still held a sacred spot in the minds of the people of Fort Wayne, and a black mark from that noble struggle would irrevocably damage the credibility of any man. Men carried their officer's rank their whole lives; Stratton felt that revelation of a dishonorable discharge should completely discredit Myers's testimony. However, true to form, Myers confronted the issue directly with the defense attorney. He readily admitted that he had initially been given a dishonorable discharge by a drunken colonel, but he explained that, when the circumstances had become known, he subsequently was honorably reinstated. He then stated that he had broken his wrist when he'd fallen from a horse and thus had been unable to enter battle. The explanation seemed to satisfy the court and the spectators. The witness was dismissed.

While Professor Myers had been expounding from the witness stand on that Wednesday, January 23, readers of the *Fort Wayne Daily News* were treated to a remarkable document that most of the city's citizens considered the college faculty's public admission of their collective guilt. Probably in response to the grand jury's declaration of them as a "public nuisance," the faculty released a copy of a faculty resolution that denounced the practice of body snatching, which had been signed by all those members who were remaining in Fort Wayne, colleagues and antagonists, including Van Buskirk and Myers.[37] The name of Professor Harold A. Clark, professor of anatomy, was conspicuous in its absence:

> WHEREAS: This community has been recently excited by body snatching and resurrections of bodies for purposes of dissection.
>
> At a meeting of the faculty of the Medical College of Fort Wayne, it was unanimously
>
> Resolved, That no dead bodies interred in any of cemetery of Allen County by the friends of the deceased, shall by our consent or connivance, be disturbed, and that we will discourage any such attempts by medical students or other persons, and further more, that we will assist in all proper efforts to punish the perpetrators of such deeds.
>
> B.S. Woodworth, MD
> C.B. Stemen, MD

---

37 *Fort Wayne Daily News*, January 23, 1878, 2.

H.D. Wood, MD
Norman Teal, MD
Thos. J. Dills, MD
F.S.C. Graveston, MD
J.L. Gilbert, MD
A.E. Van Buskirk, MD
H.V. Van Sweringen, MD
W.H. Myers, MD.

The trial resumed Thursday morning and was comically interrupted by the defense's attempt to call a woman named Hattie Orvis who had been designated to denigrate further the character of Professor Myers, though it was unclear what she might have to say. In any event, she did not appear. The police were sent to retrieve her, but they had to search her house twice before finding her hiding under a four-poster bed. After extracting her from the lair, Hattie was taken to Judge Borden's courtroom where her testimony contributed nothing to the case.

The rest of the afternoon in the circuit court consisted of a parade of defense witnesses, each testifying to the bad reputation of Professor William H. Myers. Among them was Bishop J. Dwenger, the same Bishop of St. Joseph Hospital who had confronted Professor Myers during his student lectures about his attempt to take Whitey Dan's corpse. In December, the outraged Bishop Dwenger had led the hospital's charge to expel Myers from its medical staff, and he still chafed under his failure in the endeavor. The Bishop testified that he knew Myers only too well and that his reputation "for truth and veracity" was not good. He reiterated the legal difficulties that he and the hospital had endured with the doctor.

The distinguished Dr. Isaac Rosenthal next ascended to the witness-box. As one of the co-founders of the medical college who had sat with Myers at the Aveline's salon during the hospital's founding meeting, Dr. Rosenthal admitted his dislike for Myers and affirmed that the surgeon had a poor reputation.

Next up was A.C. Nill, a druggist, who echoed the sentiments of Dr. Rosenthal.

Another witness described Myers as the "biggest liar in town."

After having denigrated the testimony of Professor Myers as best as it could, the defense returned to establish its own version of what had happened. J.Q. called the druggist William Wright, whose pharmacy occupied the first floor of the medical college building. Unrelated to the deceased Charles Wright, William Wright was in a position to know all the doctors and students at the school— after all, he saw them come and go every day because the medical college was in the same building as his store. He specified that he knew Professors Clark and Myers on sight. Therefore, he knew more than most about the night of the body snatch.

In contradiction to the story given by Professor Myers, Wright testified that he had seen Myers enter the college with Dr. Harold Clark, not Dr. Van Buskirk, on Friday afternoon November 23, the day after the burial and the day before the reward had been announced. According to the druggist, Myers and Clark had remained in the college for several hours during that day, but he could not say precisely what they had been doing. The police had arrived at the college around three o'clock that afternoon, but they hadn't been able to gain entry. According to Wright, both William Myers and Harold A. Clark had remained in the college for several hours after the police left. The druggist confirmed that he also knew Van Buskirk on sight, and that he was positive it was Clark, not Van Buskirk, who had gone into the college with Professor Myers. He estimated that Myers and Clark were there for a total of three or four hours.

After a brief cross-examination by the prosecution, which merely confirmed that Wright knew all of the professors and that he was familiar with the location of the college rooms, the pharmacist was dismissed.

Mrs. J.P. Sommers, the wife of the large student doctor known as Big Sommers (whose own trial was pending), then testified that she had been with her husband the entire evening of November 22, and that they had dined on oysters at Engleman's boarding house. They'd stayed in the dining room until about one o'clock in the morning; another student, Dr. Crooks, and Mr. Engleman had been with them. She acknowledged that her husband had been indicted on the charge of body snatching, but she swore he had been at Engleman's the entire night. She added that they had gone away for two weeks over the Christmas holidays and thus had missed the entire Justice Ryan proceedings; they had not even known that her husband had been suspected until they had returned.

After a few more character witnesses, the court was adjourned until Friday.

The trial resumed at 2:30 p.m. Friday afternoon with the testimony of the defendant, Dr. A.E. Van Buskirk. A.E. had prepared himself to speak with an assuredness that he had been unable to muster before, but the essence of his testimony was unchanged from his garbled statement to the justice of the peace. He again denied that he had gone to Lindenwood Cemetery on the night of November 22, and he swore that he never had gone to Fletcher and Powers Livery. He also denied that he was even acquainted with the manager, M.E. Woodward, until he'd met him at the last trial before Justice Ryan. A.E. then reiterated that he had never hired a wagon from there except to haul baggage or passengers to and from the railroad depot. He denied that he had paid money to Woodward that night but admitted he might have paid fees to someone at Fletcher and Powers for hauling passengers, "live ones," at some time. He denied the assertion that he and Charles Feltz were friends, and he repeated his claim that he had never gone with Feltz to any cemetery, not Lindenwood, not the Lutheran cemetery, or any other. Van Buskirk's testimony was briefly interrupted when he was asked to step outside the witness-box to allow Judge Lowry, (who had presided over the grand jury investigation) to testify briefly. Judge Lowry submitted that Dr. Myers's reputation in the city "for truth and veracity" were good. Then Dr. Van Buskirk was recalled to continue his testimony in which he described his meeting with Dr. Myers to discuss the proper approach to the police investigation, but he denied going to Lindenwood Cemetery. The defense requested he confirm his testimony to "State's counsel" that he and Feltz did not take Wright's body from Lindenwood.

The prosecutor then chose not to re-examine Van Buskirk for the time being, but he recalled the wagon driver, Charles Feltz. From the start, the case had seemed to rest on the statements of the wagon driver from the livery who had chauffeured the doctor and his students to the cemetery to pick up the body of Charles Wright. As confirmed later by the eminent I.D.G. Nelson, the grand jury foreman, and other members of the grand jury, Feltz had denied to them that he'd had any involvement; however, apparently, after being granted immunity, he now admitted his participation— which he described in great detail. According to the police chief, Feltz had admitted to him his complicity a few days after the investigation began, and Justice Ryan had granted Feltz immunity from prosecution in order to cement the case against the others.

Unfortunately, Charles Feltz apparently had interpreted his immunity as a license to tell whatever tale popped into his head. In the witness-box, he was given an opportunity again, but for some reason he seemed to feel that his continued immunity depended upon telling the most consistent and elaborate description of body-snatching events as possible. The suddenly chastened Charles Feltz now admitted that he had lied during his previous testimony before the justice of the peace about the night of November 22. Under the terms of his immunity, he now confessed that he not only had driven the doctor and the medical students to Lindenwood Cemetery that night, but that he had been driving wagons for the medical college throughout the fall to many different cemeteries. He explained that those nocturnal sojourns were a regular occurrence, and included picking up passengers at the railroad depot. Buoyed by the titillation rippling over the courtroom, the draymen smugly let it be known that he and Van Buskirk had just been to the Lutheran cemetery a night or so before the trip to Lindenwood. As Feltz stepped down, the moans of one especially distraught widow rose high above the crescendo that wafted over the crowded courtroom.

Prosecutor Robert Stratton recalled the defendant to explain these new allegations, but the anatomist was not swayed from his denials. He declared that he did not even know that there was a graveyard near the Lutheran college, nor did he know the location of the Lutheran cemetery. But Feltz's revelations had clearly rattled him. Dr. Van Buskirk did acknowledge that, in retrospect, he had been mistaken in his previous testimony; he now believed that he had, on occasion, used the Fletcher and Powers Livery to deliver passengers from the station to his home in November, but he had never hired them for any other purpose. The prosecutor again asked about the burial of Wright's head under a tree, but he reiterated his determined denial. He said that they always used an old coal barrel at the school to deposit discarded flesh from the cadavers.

The doctor was clearly upset that Prosecutor Robert Stratton's macabre questions about disposing of the head had come on the heels of Feltz's testimony. So the prosecutor pressed his advantage and got A.E. to admit he'd become concerned when he'd heard about the Lindenwood episode, and that he, in fact, had met with Myers and Clark, as described by Professor Myers. He affirmed that they'd met at the contractor Myers's home. He also confirmed Myers's testimony about going back to the school and finding it surrounded by the constabulary, but he did not admit to going back later with Myers to dissect the body, as the surgeon had claimed and as the druggist, Wright, had contradicted. Van Buskirk readily acknowledged that he procured anatomical subjects for the school, but he insisted that they were shipped into Fort Wayne by freight and not through Fletcher and Powers. He described how the school sold the bodies to the students at $4 each, with five students assigned to one cadaver. He denied that he had gone to the medical college the night of November 23, and denied that he had testified otherwise before Justice Ryan. At that point, the emotionally spent Van Buskirk slouched in his chair and was asked to step down.

Next, Mr. Isaac De Groff Nelson, president of Lindenwood Cemetery, strode to the front of the courtroom. Coincidentally, Nelson had been serving as foreman of the grand jury and, in that capacity, he had investigated the body snatching and, later, had indicted Van Buskirk. He described to the prosecutor how Van Buskirk had testified at the December grand jury's investigation. He confirmed Feltz's testimony that Dr. Van Buskirk had not been interviewed until well after the jury had heard from the wagon driver. Nelson said that, to the best of his recollection, at the time of the grand jury investigation, Charles Feltz had not even mentioned Dr. Van Buskirk's name, nor had anyone else. He added that Feltz had begun to arouse the grand jury's suspicion about his own possible role when he falsely claimed to have been delivering passengers for Fletcher and Powers that night. Nelson knew that Feltz had already admitted his involvement in the drive to Lindenwood when the chief of police had questioned him in November, just after news of the affair had broken. Then, at the more recent grand jury hearing for the present circuit court proceeding, Feltz had changed his story again and admitted that he had gone to Lindenwood that night. Nelson further testified, at that second grand jury before the present trial, that Feltz had admitted that, in fact, he had driven a delivery wagon with Van Buskirk, Big Sommers, and others, though he wasn't sure about the exact number of his passengers. He'd also described picking up the body and riding back with the doctors to the medical college.

Prosecutor Robert Stratton then asked Mr. Nelson what he knew about Professor Myers. Nelson testified that he knew Myers and that his reputation for truth and veracity was good, except for his troubles with the doctors. On cross-examination, Nelson asserted that Myers's difficulties were entirely with the doctors, but then added that he was known around the city of Fort Wayne for not paying his debts. Nelson then remembered that, at the first grand jury sessions, Dr. Hiram Van Sweringen, Myers's brother-in-law, had been asked to deliver a complete list of the faculty at the college of medicine, but he had not known if the doctor had ever completed that task.

Finally, the prosecutor asked Nelson about his relationship with Chief Diehl. He responded that he had discussed the case with the police chief but that there had been no conversation about the reward.

The prosecutor then called Police Chief Hugh Diehl to the stand. The chief described his investigation of the crime. He stated that though the law was limited in what it could do in cases of body snatching even with convictions, the broad community outrage, combined with Lindenwood's offer of the reward, had required his sharpest attention. He testified that after the reward was offered on November 24, he and his assistant, Police Lieutenant Frank Wilkinson, had gone to the medical college around one o'clock in the afternoon and had searched all the rooms, except the dissection laboratory because it had been locked. He said that Dr. Crooks, one of the medical students, had barred their entry to the chamber. After leaving the medical college, they'd gone immediately to Dr. Myers's office to discuss the matter with him. The chief vigorously denied that he had made an arrangement with Myers, or with any of the other witnesses, including Feltz and Pantlind. He conceded that he wanted the $1,000 reward as much as anyone and, in the re-direct, Diehl admitted that it had required the purchase of a few beers to get Pantlind to tell what he knew about the matter. (At that point, Van Buskirk's attorney, J.Q. Stratton, interjected that Pantlind drinks almost as much beer as much as the witness, Chief Diehl!) The chief heatedly dismissed Prosecutor Stratton's assertion that he had made an arrangement with Myers whereby Clark and Myers would reveal the perpetrator's name in such a manner that Diehl could serendipitously overhear their conversation as evidence against Van Buskirk. The chief assured the court that it was natural for him to have gone to Professor Myers for an explanation about what might have happened because Myers was so well known in the city that he had become the de facto spokesperson for the school, regardless of its internal administrative organization.

One interesting witness was Mr. Edwin Evans who lived on the second floor, across the street from the medical college. Evans testified that he had been awakened around two o'clock the morning of November 22, perhaps by the crunching of wagon wheels on the pavement. He glanced across the street to investigate and was struck by what he described as the unusual appearance of light emanating from upper floor windows of the medical college on Broadway. Evans must not have been paying much attention on other nights because it was common for medical students to dissect all night long.

Finally, the prosecution seemed to have felt compelled to rectify the aspersions cast by the myriad of character witnesses against their key witness, William H. Myers. They called forth a succession of gentlemen who testified to the fine reputation of Professor Myers. As noted, earlier in the day, Dr. Van Buskirk had been asked to step down temporarily in order to hear the character testimony of another judge, Judge Lowry, who was available to testify on behalf of Professor Myers. He stated that he had never heard Myers's character questioned, that his reputation for truth was good. Then came a fresh array of individuals to present their own version of Lowry's ennobling description of the surgeon. The most prominent was the venerable Colonel Robertson who admitted that he was also Myers's attorney.

The evidence against the anatomist appeared to be overwhelming. The wagon driver, Charles Feltz; Feltz's colleague, Henry Pantlind; and the livery manager, Woodward, all had testified that Van Buskirk had ordered the wagon and had ridden in it with Feltz and some medical students to Lindenwood Cemetery, and that they all had returned in the wagon that then carried a body bound for the medical college. The testimonies of Professor W.H. Myers; his son the medical student, Herschel Myers; and the neighbor, Edwin Evans, all seemed to have forged an unbreakable chain between the body theft, the demonstrator of anatomy, and the predawn dissection in the college's third floor rooms. The defense consisted mainly of Van Buskirk's denial that, though it admittedly had improved on the second repetition, remained unconvincing; the inconsistencies in the testimonies of some of the prosecution witnesses; and the parade of disputations of Professor Myers's character. (The latter had been refuted by an impressive rank of respected citizens who testified on behalf of the surgeon.)

Discrediting the prevaricating drayman, Charles Feltz, posed a less daunting task to the defense, because the wagon driver's story had shifted with the winds through the courtroom, and he admitted that he had lied.

No one could anticipate any verdict but guilty. In the street outside, wagers ran so strongly against Van Buskirk that, despite the many offers, no one would bet against conviction at any odds.

Someone should have taken that bet.

For the jury, the matter had become far murkier than community sentiment suggested. Judge Borden had instructed the members of the jury to consider only the testimony brought before the court in regard to the matter of the body snatching at Lindenwood. Further, they were specifically told that in their deliberations, they must disregard the statements given by the wagon driver, Charles Feltz, and the professor of surgery, William H. Myers, because they had lied in their testimony.

The bewildered jurors deliberated for twenty-two hours until the following morning. They faced a daunting proposition. Their friends and neighbors in the city of Fort Wayne had no doubt about Van Buskirk's involvement in stealing Wright's body and ached for his conviction to bring the matter to its rightful close. After all, it was literally his job to procure bodies. The newspapers asked: "If Van Buskirk didn't steal Wright's body, who did?"[38]

Other issues made the jury's decision difficult. The college faculty effectively had publicly admitted their guilt with their signed resolution. To compound the effrontery, Feltz had reported that the Wright robbery was just one of many. Even as the trial wound to a close, the distraught widow of Diedrich Buck beseeched the Lutheran cemetery to investigate her husband's grave. In addition, the townspeople continued to worry about the ghouls who they felt still must have been lurking around the city. The newspaper announced that the grave of Mathis Stodel, who had died while the trial was taking place, would be heavily guarded throughout the night. But, the jury could not take any of that into account. They were to consider only the evidence before them.

But because the now impeached testimonies of Feltz and Myers would have comprised the principal evidence against the anatomist, no one should have been surprised when the jury returned to the circuit court room around one o'clock in the afternoon of Monday, January 28, with a verdict of "not guilty." As Bessie Van Buskirk had told my father, the bells of the courthouse tolled Van Buskirk's acquittal. The people of Fort Wayne were appalled, but the headlines read: "Van Buskirk is Happy."[39]

---

38 *Fort Wayne Daily News*, January 28, 1878.
39 *Fort Wayne Daily News*, January 28, 1878.

Members of the jury later confessed that they had had little doubt about the guilt of the accused, but without the testimony of Feltz and Myers, there simply was insufficient evidence presented in the courtroom to convict the doctor.

CHAPTER 14

The Buck Business

VAN BUSKIRK MIGHT HAVE BEEN "happy" about his acquittal, but he surely knew that his problems were far from over. Although the testimony of the wagon driver, Charles Feltz, had been impeached from consideration by the jury, the people in the courtroom had heard his tales. Feltz's implication of the doctors from the medical college in the robbing of local graves had become more and more believable as the trial had progressed. He finally admitted that not only had he driven Van Buskirk and the other doctors to Lindenwood on the night of November 22, but also that the particular midnight drive to Lindenwood had followed on the heels of many more that had been taking place on a regular basis while the college was in session. His depiction of another trip to Emanuel Lutheran Cemetery two nights earlier struck a horrific chord for the widow, Sophia Buck. Feltz had described the day and the place she had buried her husband, Diedrich.

Even as the prosecution closed their arguments in the case of A.E. Van Buskirk for the stealing of Charles Wright's body, Sophia Buck demanded an investigation of her husband's gravesite. By Saturday, January 26, Police Chief Hugh Diehl and his officers had acquired the pertinent documents to oversee the raising of Diedrich Buck's coffin. They weren't surprised to find the familiar splintered fracture that extended through its lid from one side to the other, about a third of the distance between the head and foot. The lid was lifted; the box was empty except for the sepulchral clothing. Sophia Buck became so "perfectly wild" at the graveside that she needed to be restrained. She was taken home amid speculation that her mind would never recover.

The widow Buck did, however, regain her senses to testify against the arrested perpetrators. Sophia Buck lived another four decades to the age of 94. Her obituary made no mention of the travesty that surrounded her husband's grave, only that her husband Diedrich had preceded her in death by some forty-five years. Horrified as she had been by the discovery, Sophia Buck was not completely surprised that her husband's body had been taken. Even at the time of his funeral, she had been terribly concerned about the possibility; every new widow in Fort Wayne worried about the same. Like Mary Wright's misplaced confidence in the sanctity of Lindenwood, Sophia Buck had believed that burial in the Emanuel Lutheran Cemetery would offer a modicum of protection. Feltz had claimed that those November trips to Lindenwood and Emanuel Lutheran were the only ones they had taken to those particular graveyards, but no one really believed his disclaimers.

Although the discovery of the robbing of Buck's grave had occurred as a consequence of the Wright trial and coincided with the closing arguments, the new information about Buck could not be considered as evidence against Van Buskirk. By the time Buck's empty coffin was discovered, the Wright jury had been preparing for its deliberations to determine whether or not Dr. Van Buskirk should be held accountable for the resurrection of Charles Wright, not of Diedrich Buck. That would come later.

As the jury began to consider the Wright case on Monday, January 28, everyone in Fort Wayne already knew about the robbing of Buck's grave, which only fueled their conviction that the anatomist was guilty. The unexpected acquittal stirred the cauldron of communal fury to the boiling point. Lutheran congregations held "indignation meetings" to express their umbrage over the occurrence and their sorrow for both the Wright and the Buck families.[40] They prayed for everyone involved. Now it was the Lutheran Board of Trustees' turn to meet, but they had no need to offer a reward. The perpetrator was already known. He had escaped two trials—one before the justice of the peace, the other at the county court—for the heinous crimes, but he would not skirt a third.

The Buck case had seemed clear-cut from the beginning. The revelation of Diedrich Buck's empty coffin had lent credence to the earlier impeached and disregarded testimony of the wagon driver, Charles Feltz, and it compounded the communal anger toward the medical college. Tuesday's newspaper announced the acquittal with the observation that though the jury had found Van Buskirk not guilty, the public had no doubt that he had done it. One editor even went so far as to propose that Police Chief Diehl be granted at least part of the Lindenwood reward because he had tracked down the criminal and brought him to trial. They felt that Diehl should not be penalized because the demonstrator had managed to slip through a legal loophole.

The following day, the papers blamed the entire medical college for the horror that now permeated the city of Fort Wayne. It was true that many of the college doctors had testified in Van Buskirk's defense. Even the outspoken Professor Myers, Van Buskirk's principal antagonist, publicly defended the practice of grave robbing as a necessity to provide subject material for medical students. However, the *Daily News* asserted that the medical college "has forfeited every claim to respect." The reporting observed that the railroad shopmen didn't "take much stock" in the medical college, which was a damning development considering that the railroads employed many of the Fort Wayne workers. The collective attitude of the shopmen was a bellwether for community sentiment. Several

---

40 *Fort Wayne Daily Sentinel*, January 28, 1878, 4.

of the college doctors had contracts as surgeons with the railroad companies to treat the many train injuries.

By the end of the week, the people of Fort Wayne had turned their umbrage from the Wright debacle to the stealing of Diedrich Buck's body. The newspapers of Friday, February 1, complained that no action had been yet taken. By Monday, the editors wondered if the whole Buck affair simply had been dropped.

In addition, some of the doctors were already threatening to leave the Medical College of Fort Wayne. They discussed starting a new medical school whose first order would be to garner public support. William Myers, never a wallflower, already had resigned from his position as professor of surgery. Despite the many internal confrontations with Myers, his resignation had cut deeply into an already mortally wounded school. Considering the chasm left with Myers's departure, the faculty's choice of his successor, a medical student, was all the more strange: Dr. W.T. Atkins from Chicago would graduate from the Fort Wayne college the following month. Although his achievement to become his class valedictorian might had been impressive, it hardly qualified him to assume his distinguished professor's leadership position on the faculty. Some wondered if perhaps the appointment signaled a collective recognition that the days of the school were numbered. Van Buskirk's prediction about Myers's nefarious motivations toward the institution seemed to be coming to fruition.

Despite the almost daily scandals among the doctors, the business of medicine proceeded in Fort Wayne because people continued to require medical help. On Wednesday, the same newspaper that had impugned Dr. Myers and the college of medicine as public nuisances extolled the surgeon Myers's excision of a decayed foot bone from a young man in his parents' home. Amid the public turmoil and resentment swirling about, the medical college also had its own mundane business to conduct. Classes concluded for the academic year, and the school scheduled its commencement for

Wednesday, February 20. On February 6, the *Daily News* ran an announcement that the "Fort Wayne Institute of Body Snatching" would hold its graduation ceremony at the Methodist church.[41] The church must have had a change of heart about hosting its unsavory neighbor, for a few days later, the event was rescheduled at "The Rink," a public, secular auditorium, officially named "The People's Theatre." It held a popular skating rink. (*See Fig. 11.*) The commencement exercises proceeded without any untoward events. The Reverend Moffit gave the address, and Dr. Myers's successor, W.T. Atkins, soon to be professor of surgery, gave the valedictory speech.

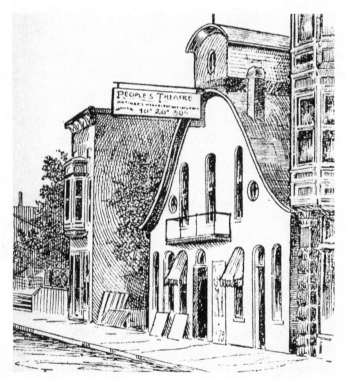

Figure 11. Fort Wayne's People's Theatre, locally known as "The Rink" for its large and popular skating rink, was also used for public lectures and other events.[42]

41 *Fort Wayne Daily News*, February 6, 1878.

42 John Akenbruck, *The Fort Wayne Story* (Woodland Hills, CA: Windsor Publications, 1980).

Professor Myers attended the commencement ceremonies and commented that the future of the school looked bright, at least financially. Since he had been so personally involved in the college's ultimate fate, the professor surely knew otherwise.

On Thursday, February 7, the grand jury indicted Dr. A.E. Van Buskirk for robbing the grave of Diedrich Buck on November 19 of the previous year. Bail was set at $1,000. The student, Jacob B. Sommers, known as Big Sommers, who had been unavailable during the first trials, also was indicted for stealing the body of Charles Wright. Two months later, on April 6, those indictments were expanded to include Sommers as well as Van Buskirk for the Diedrich Buck affair.

Big Sommers was a practical man. He had already established a modest local medical practice, undoubtedly like many of his classmates, on the basis of a medical preceptorship. He merely wanted to complete his academic medical training to qualify for a doctor of medicine degree and get back to his practice, his future thus assured. By then, he had been able to see the turmoil to which Dr. Van Buskirk had subjected himself by fighting the charges. After all, as the surgeon William T. Myers allegedly had explained to the demonstrator shortly after the snatch was discovered, legally, body snatching was a relatively minor crime, a misdemeanor that usually carried a modest fine. Sommers promptly pleaded guilty to both charges. He paid the minimal fine of $25, as predicted months before by Professor Myers. Big Sommers never underwent a protracted trial. He simply paid what he owed and stepped off the legal stage and out of the limelight.

But A.E. fought on. His attorneys filed a petition for a change of venue with Judge Borden. The request was denied, but the judge seemed to have had his fill of the grave robbers and willingly turned the case over to another judge. People of Fort Wayne began to doubt if Van Buskirk would ever be tried for the Buck robbery, but, much to the disappointment of the defendant, a new judge was promptly assigned to his case. That time it was Judge Lowry, the same Judge Lowry who was a close friend of Professor Myers and who had testified for the prosecution during Van Buskirk's previous trial. To compound the demonstrator's foreboding, Samuel Hench, the attorney who the Lindenwood board had unsuccessfully petitioned to prosecute the Wright case, now agreed to prosecute in the Buck trial.

The weeks crept by from winter to spring, and the public chafed for resolution. April trial dates came and passed after repeated postponements. Jury selection dragged on longer than expected but, finally, the trial was set for May 20, 1878. As the court convened that Monday, the prosecution was forced to request another delay because one of the witnesses, a traveling salesman named Arthur Dodge, had left town and was not available. Judge Lowry postponed the trial for one more week with the hope of locating Dodge.

The following Monday, May 27, Lowry reconvened his court. The jury was in place and the witnesses were assembled, including the unrepentant Arthur Dodge. Judge Lowry instructed his jury. He warned the participants and the spectators that the court would tolerate no diversions or prevarications. He announced his intention to proceed with prudence but toward a swift conclusion; he declared that he wanted to complete the trial by Thursday of that same week and that he would hold evening sessions if necessary to meet that deadline. The judge then adjourned until four o'clock that afternoon.

The first and only witnesses for that first evening session were the widow, Sophia Buck, who was by then fully recovered from her swoon, and her twenty-year-old son, Charles. They described the graveside service and the location of Diedrich's grave. Apparently, Mrs. Buck had not noticed a newcomer who had joined the procession of mourners in their cortege to the cemetery, but it wasn't uncommon for strangers to take an interest in public funeral services. The widow testified that her husband's feet were deformed with the toes lapped under each other and also that he had had a "rupture." Her son added that his father was about five feet eight inches tall and bearded. The court was adjourned until nine o'clock on Tuesday morning when they would hear from the notorious drayman, Charles Feltz.

Early the following morning, witnesses, reporters, and onlookers found themselves in close quarters again, but that time on a hot day in late spring. Humid Indiana air clung to spectators like moss on a rotting stump. A sweaty Charles Feltz took the stand promptly as scheduled. His eyes darted around the room as if they were seeking a safe place to rest, but he pulled himself together as his testimony gathered steam.

Feltz explained that on November 19, Dr. Van Buskirk from the medical college had come to Fletcher and Powers to reserve a wagon for that same evening. The driver added that, later, the doctor returned to the livery for the rig and driver. He had even helped the drayman hitch the team to the wagon, and then the two of them had set out in the direction of Emanuel Lutheran Cemetery on Maumee Road. As they approached the graveyard, Van Buskirk ordered him to stop in a low ravine where three men were awaiting their arrival—Big Sommers and two others whom he didn't know. From his seat on the wagon, Feltz said he could see a long sack lying inside the graveyard, leaning against the wrought iron bars. It could have contained a body, but, of course, he could not see inside. The senior doctor climbed off the wagon and, along with the three men, retrieved the sack and loaded it onto the wagon. The doctor then sat beside the driver again and that time instructed him to head back toward town along Wayne Street to the home of Professor Myers where Big Sommers disembarked. They then proceeded back to the medical college on the corner of Washington and Broadway. As his passengers lugged their awkward load into the building's side door, Feltz returned to his stables.

The prosecution next called Mr. M.E. Woodward, the manager of the Fletcher and Powers Livery. Woodward, who had also testified in the Wright trial, recalled that a young man had come to the stables on the afternoon of Monday, November 19, to inquire about a wagon and team for later that night. He had made no specific arrangements, but he wanted to be sure that a wagon would be available, if needed. He had said that if the wagon was called for, Dr. Van Buskirk would pay. Woodward remembered that, some days later, Van Buskirk did come to pay for livery services. The stable manager had given the same testimony in the Wright case; perhaps the interval of several months had confused his recollection of the specific payments. Woodward couldn't remember the precise day that Van Buskirk had paid, but he did remember leaving orders specifically for Charles Feltz to drive the wagon if the doctors needed it. Woodward sat down.

Prosecutor Hench next called the bombastic Dr. William H. Myers who had managed thus far, despite impeachment of his previous testimony, to implicate Van Buskirk and to extricate himself from blame. At the same time, Myers had sufficiently disrupted the medical college so that it had been brought to the brink of collapse. Myers himself hinted about a second medical college that would be known as the Fort Wayne Medical College, which, indeed, was to come to fruition even as the trial proceeded.

As the new trial proceeded, Myers testified that on November 20, Van Buskirk had spoken with him in the faculty room on the third floor of the medical college. Van Buskirk had asked him if he planned to go out to the Lutheran cemetery. Myers claimed to have denied any such plans but iterated that Van Buskirk had told him that he didn't wish the professor to dig into an empty grave, because he had been there the night before and had taken the body. Feltz's testimony that Big Sommers had disembarked at Myers's house strongly implicated Myers's immediate knowledge of the affair, but the surgeon persisted, confident that he would be taken at his word. Eloquent as he was, it was difficult for anyone who had followed the trials to believe that he had not known exactly what was taking place. Professor Myers continued his testimony with the claim that he was not in the dissecting room on November 21, but, as he had testified before, he had been there with Van Buskirk a few nights later when Charles Wright's body had been dissected. Myers reported that he had noticed Buck's body on another table at the time, distinctive because of the severe deformation of the second toe on the left foot. He recalled that he had taken a bone chisel himself and had amputated what became headlined as "The Tell Tale Toe."[43] In addition, Myers pointed out that Dr. Van Buskirk had drawn his attention to the subject's inconsequential right inguinal hernia. Defense Attorney Stratton's cross-examination failed to dent Myers's testimony. The prosecution then recalled Sophia Buck who did remember seeing Big Sommers at her husband's funeral, but said that she hadn't thought much about it at the time. The Sommers' were neighbors; it was natural that he would have attended Diedrich's funeral. Young Charles Buck concurred, and the state rested its case.

The defense then rose to call that same procession of medical students who were intensely loyal to their demonstrator of anatomy. Dr. Crooks—the same doctor who had barred Chief Diehl's entry to the dissection laboratory back in December—testified that he was in the laboratory working every night from November 14 through December, and that he never saw any corpse with deformed feet nor did he recall seeing one that was "ruptured." In cross-examination, Crooks claimed that he had dissected four or five corpses during that time.

Two other students, Lipes and Ruhl, concurred with Crooks.

Three other community physicians who had part-time appointments at the medical college—including Hiram Van

---

43 *Fort Wayne Daily News*, January 28, 1878.

Sweringen, William Myers's brother-in-law—supported the students' testimonies.

Van Sweringen, the venerable Dr. Woodworth, the disgruntled ex-prisoners, Drs. Buchman and Dills, and several others in succession all agreed that Professor Myers was a known liar whose testimony could not be trusted.

The defense then recalled the members of the December grand jury, all of whom agreed that Feltz had never implicated Van Buskirk until he was granted his own immunity. Although Big Sommers had already admitted his guilt, no one other than the prevaricating Feltz had actually testified that Dr. Van Buskirk personally had been to Buck's grave.

Other witnesses followed, including Dr. Woods, who claimed he knew Big Sommers well, and that he had seen Sommers and another student, Sledd, go into a saloon on the night of November 19. And when Mr. John Clive, a member of the grand jury, testified, he said that when Feltz finally did admit to his involvement in the Wright affair, he had added that it was the only body snatching with which he had ever been involved.

Thus, the defense attorney felt he had instilled enough doubt about the veracity of key witnesses that Van Buskirk could safely claim his innocence.

A weary Dr. A.E. Van Buskirk then rose to testify on his own behalf, but both he and the court appeared to be spent. A.E. had been fighting these charges against him for over six months, merely for doing his job. It was clear he did not have much fight left in him, and he probably wondered if he should have taken Myers's advice back then to simply admit his actions and move on. Nonetheless, Van Buskirk once again took his place on the witness stand and, in response to direct questions from his attorney, simply denied everything heinous.

He did admit that he was responsible for procuring cadavers. On the other hand, he denied going to Fletcher and Powers and to the cemetery. He claimed that he had gone directly home around nine o'clock on the evening of November 19. He denied any conversation with Myers about Diedrich Buck and said he could not recall any cadavers with deformed feet or even with a hernia. In cross-examination, the doctor admitted that "to some extent" it was his duty to "furnish subjects for the use of students," and that he supposed they had dissected about nine during the fall term.

After a brief recess followed by more testimony to the bad reputation of Professor Myers, the defense rested.

Irritating as he must have been to many of his former colleagues, Myers was never one to shrink from controversy. Just two days after his testimony in the contentious trial of Dr. Van Buskirk, even as the jury was considering A.E.'s verdict, Professor Myers was emboldened to present a public lecture that evening at "The Rink" entitled "Resurrection and the Dead." To the disappointment of about 200 people in his audience, Myers refused to allude to Van Buskirk or to anyone concerning the body-snatching cases that had recently transfixed the city. Instead, he delivered a scholarly dissertation on ancient and modern views of the dead, the advances in the study of anatomy, and the importance of anatomic dissection for the training of good doctors. Echoing the query of the British anatomist Sir Astley Cooper fifty years earlier, Myers said he wondered how a person who would not entrust his watch to an inexperienced watchmaker would entrust his infinitely more complex body to someone who had never taken one apart.

During the questioning period following his lecture, Myers refused to discuss the current case before the jury. He did not hesitate to describe his own exploits in the Van Wert, Ohio, graveyard sometime before, and the more recent Whitey Dan affair. As often occurred when Myers spoke, the audience wondered which parts were true.

Back in the courtroom, in rebuttal to the litany of testaments to Myers's evil reputation, the state presented an equally long and undoubtedly more prominent list of witnesses who testified on behalf of the former professor of surgery. Judge Lowry denied the state's request that the guilty plea of Big Sommers for the same crime be entered into the court record.

True to his word, Judge Lowry managed to steer the prosecution and defense through the Diedrich Buck's trial to completion by Thursday evening. Prosecutor Hench and defense attorney J.Q. Stratton each spoke for about an hour either against or in support of the defendant; final arguments concluded at 9:30 p.m. The judge charged the jury and sent them off to deliberate; he hadn't given them much time, for it was nearly ten o'clock when they began. They were all tired and cranky, but no one expected the verdict to take long. On the face of it, it came down to Van Buskirk's bald denial of his involvement against the detailed description of the events of November 19 as provided by the wagon driver, Charles Feltz. That time, however, Feltz's testimony was admitted for the jury's consideration, as was that of Professor Myers, who was concluding his lecture on the importance of anatomy as the jury began its discussion.

Although many people who worked closely with the bombastic surgeon found him self-centered and untrustworthy, the favorable testimony by many of Fort Wayne's most prominent citizens nullified the defense's attempts to discount the crusty surgeon.

The jury missed Judge Lowry's deadline by only one hour. At one o'clock in the morning of Friday, May 31, 1878, the jury announced it had reached its verdict: they found A.E. Van Buskirk guilty. They recommended a fine of $400 and court costs amounting to an additional $150. Later, it was learned that the jury had had no doubt about his guilt and had voted unanimously on the first ballot. The remainder of the time had been spent debating the amount of fine to be assessed. Opinions had wavered between the minimum $25 that Sommers had already paid after his admission of guilt and the maximum of $1,000. The editor of the newspaper could not resist the comment that the anatomist could have acquired sixteen stiffs at $25 each for the $400 he paid.

Although Van Buskirk was no doubt resigned to his fate, his attorney, J.Q. Stratton, immediately moved for a new trial. Judge Lowry, however, overruled the motion. He agreed with the jury's verdict and assessed the fine. Van Buskirk gave "replevin bail"—a promissory note to cover the fine and cost. A friend, Mr. H.C. Hartman, another attorney in Fort Wayne, provided surety to cover A.E.'s fines.

At least the long ordeal seemed to be over for both the defendant and the people of Fort Wayne. The conviction had finally come, though with punishment only in the form of a fine and freedom for the doctor, freedom to return to his work, perhaps even to his midnight sojourns. The people of Fort Wayne must have retired that Friday evening relieved, at least, that the scandal was out in the open. Few of them could have known that a resurrection in their neighboring state would change the business forever. On Saturday, June 1, they awakened to news that Van Buskirk's case had suddenly been dwarfed by a deluge of headlines extolling a far more spectacular body snatch in Ohio: The body of John Scott Harrison, son of former U.S. President William Henry Harrison, had been stolen from its heavily fortified grave in North Bend, Ohio. Body snatching would never be the same.

CHAPTER 15

A Bad Year for Resurrection

VERNIGHT, Fort Wayne's sensational body-snatching trial had dwindled to a mere footnote on the far bigger story emanating from Cincinnati. The events began some months before and foretold the end of the resurrectionists.

In January 1878, authorities of Toledo, Ohio, captured Dr. Henri Le Caron, alias Dr. Charles O. Morton, the most notorious body snatcher of northern Ohio. Le Caron had graduated from the Detroit Medical College in 1872, but he never saw many patients, at least not live ones.[44] Instead, he lurked on the dark fringes of medicine with the carny hucksters and purveyors of fresh cadavers. Le Caron had financed his medical studies by moonlighting as a body snatcher, unearthing his wares from a cemetery near Sandwich, Ontario, Canada, before selling them to medical colleges in Michigan. He found that the resurrectionist business was better suited to his talents than legitimate medical practice.

It wasn't the first time Le Caron had been apprehended, and his detention was typically brief. That January, then using the alias Dr. Charles O. Morton, Le Caron was arrested and charged with stealing two bodies from a Toledo graveyard and shipping them in pickle barrels to Ann Arbor, Michigan. Soon after his incarceration

---

44 Detroit Medical College was the forerunner to the contemporary Wayne State University School of Medicine.

in the county jail, the prisoner complained that he was severely ill. A local doctor found Le Caron to be feverish and covered with pustular, suppurative, eruptions. Fearing that the prisoner carried smallpox, there was nothing to do but transfer the inmate to the "Pest House." But soon, as the warders sat down to their supper, the pustular Henri Le Caron alias, Dr. Charles Morton—despite being overseen by two guards—slipped away into the winter's night. Later, the examining physician discovered an open bottle of croton oil that Morton must have applied to induce his dermatologic malady. Extracted from seeds of the southeast Asian croton tiglium tree, croton oil had been long used as a powerful purgative. Topically applied, croton oil was known to cause a painful, blistering rash. By 1878, the toxicity of the oil had driven the substance into medical disfavor, but the enterprising Dr. Morton must have retained a quantity for such eventualities. It would not be the last adventure of Le Caron, alias Morton. Who else could have managed Ohio's most notorious resurrection at the end of May in 1878?

Congressman John Scott Harrison, the son of the ninth president of the United States, William Henry Harrison (1773–1841), had died just north of Cincinnati on May 25, 1878. He was to be buried in the family plot at nearby North Bend, Ohio. In a chapel established by his father, the funeral service overflowed with prominent residents, for the Harrison family was among Cincinnati's most admired and beloved. John Scott's two sons, General Benjamin Harrison (who would later become president himself), and his younger brother, John, had carefully planned the entire proceedings. They, and everyone else at the funeral, knew that Charles O. Morton was still at large and that body snatching was rampant in the area. The Harrison brothers thus took extreme precautions to prevent violation of the tomb, arranging for John Scott's grave to be dug especially deep and broad, lined at the bottom and sides with heavy brick. The day before the actual funeral, John Scott's heavy coffin was lowered; three large stones weighing nearly a ton were placed on top, the largest at the head and two smaller bar-shaped blocks at the foot. Over that, a layer of cement was poured.

The grave was left open overnight for the cement to dry, but a guard was posted. The following day, nearly a ton of soil was poured over the dried cement.

But at the start of the graveside service, as the Harrison brothers walked to join the mourners, they noticed an ominous disturbance of the soil over the nearby grave, that of their nephew, Augustus Devin, a young man who had died a few days earlier. They hoped the roughened earth could be attributed to the rooting of pigs from a neighboring farm, but there was not time to investigate; the service for John Scott must go on.

After the funeral, Benjamin Harrison and his wife departed by train for Indianapolis while his younger brother, John, remained in Cincinnati. Coincidentally, the Devin family had also noticed the suspicious disarray of the soil over their son's grave. They immediately contacted the authorities, who arranged for an exhumation of Augustus's tomb. Their worst fear was confirmed: The casket was empty; Augustus Devin's body had been stolen.

John Harrison agreed to help and, along with the local constabulary, obtained a search warrant to investigate the medical colleges. They began with the most prestigious, the Medical College of Ohio. With the assistance of a reluctant janitor, they scoured each room but found no evidence of the young man's stolen body. As they were about to depart, one of the men noticed a taught rope suspended from a pulley over a dark chute. Harrison ordered the rope drawn forth. To his horror, it revealed hanging ignominiously from its end, not the body of Augustus Devin, but the naked corpse of Harrison's own father and namesake, John Scott Harrison.

Naturally, Morton, alias Le Caron (and a host of other aliases), leapt to the top of the suspect list. His work had already seemed evident in the disappearance of the body of the Harrison cousin,

Augustus Devin. Despite the intense investigation, the means of
the Harrison body snatch was never precisely determined nor was a
perpetrator ever arrested. However, it had been noted by some late
night revelers that a cart had stopped briefly in an alley alongside
the Medical College of Ohio at the door through which the school
received cadavers for anatomic dissection.

Although the focus of the investigation of the Devin case
had quickly shifted to "The Harrison Horror," the discovery
of Harrison's body at the Medical College of Ohio led police
to intensify their search for Devin's body in one of Cincinnati's
five other medical schools.[45] In the course of those inquiries, the
investigators learned that the janitor at the Miami Medical College
had been allowing "Dr. Morton" to hide his bodies in their college
morgue while he arranged their disposition. Periodically, Morton
would arrive, pack the cadavers in pickle barrels and ship them to
"Quimby and Co., Ann Arbor, Michigan." In response to this news,
the Cincinnati investigating officers embarked on the next train to
Ann Arbor where they demanded that they be allowed to inspect
the anatomical laboratory at the University of Michigan. There,
lying upon one of the Michigan dissection tables, they found the
partially dismembered corpse of young Augustus Devin.

In retrospect, it seemed likely that Harrison's interment had
been the day before his funeral, with the cement poured and allowed
to dry overnight. However, his body had been exhumed before the
cement had had time to dry. When the officers inspected the grave,
they found the two smaller stones turned upright and the coffin
lid fractured in the traditional manner. The resurrectionist or his
accomplices must have made arrangements to transport the body
directly to the Medical College of Ohio. One account suggested
that the Miami medical students might have done it to embarrass
their rival school, but that was never confirmed. It doesn't seem

---

45 Harry J Sievers, "The Harrison Horror," prepared by the Staff of the Public Library of
Fort Wayne and Allen County, 1956.

that there would have been time for the resurrectionist to deliver the body to one school, and for the students to then transfer it to the other. Furthermore, the Medical College of Ohio admitted that it had an ongoing contract with Morton, as did other schools in the city, to provide cadavers for their dissection room.[46] In the end, the grand jury indicted Morton for taking the bodies of both men, but it does not seem that he was apprehended. "Dr. Morton" had escaped again.

The events surrounding "The Harrison Horror" might have eclipsed headlines about Fort Wayne's own "resurrections," but they brought the whole business of body snatching to the forefront of America's political agenda. Headlines blasted the Harrison story from front pages across the country. On May 31, 1878, the *New York Times* ran: "Students Stealing Corpses" under "The Graveyard Robberies"; the article proclaimed that if medical colleges had no means to obtain dissection subjects other that robbing graves, they should discontinue performing anatomic dissections altogether.

It wasn't that stealing bodies was really anything new for Cincinnatians. With six different colleges of medicine and six different anatomy laboratories to satisfy, the demand for subjects always ran high. Townspeople in places like Cincinnati, Fort Wayne, Baltimore, New York, or any city with a medical college within or nearby had worried about their dead for many years. The new aspect was that now it had become undeniable that no body, not even the son of a president of the United States, was exempt. Something had to be done. Like the crafty antagonist in Arthur Conan Doyle's Sherlock Holmes short story "The Adventure of the Norwood Builder," Morton lacked "that supreme gift of the artist, the knowledge of when to stop."[47] The intense public indignation over

---

46 Suzanne M. Shultz, *Body Snatching: The Robbing of Graves for the Education of Physicians in Early Nineteenth Century America* (Jefferson, North Carolina and London: McFarland and Company, 2005).

47 Arthur C. Doyle, *The Return of Sherlock Holmes* (London: Georges Newnes, Ltd., 1905).

the Harrison snatch cast a public spotlight on the resurrectionists that did not fade and could not be extinguished. By its glow, the resurrectionists could see that their days were numbered. Perhaps Dr. Morton just couldn't restrain himself from taking the corpse of a president's son. Until that time, most body thefts either had gone entirely undetected or had incited a short-lived local scandal that dwindled until the next one occurred. Indeed, if it were not for the investigation of the Devin case, even the theft of John Scott Harrison's body may never have been detected. By the same token, no one would ever have known about the resurrection of Fort Wayne's Diedrich Buck had not the wagon driver mentioned it during the Wright trial. It was true that the resurrectionists generally preferred bodies from the potter's field or of migrants who didn't have friends and loved ones nearby to complain.

Of course, by then most people knew that body thieves foraged well beyond the potter's fields, but perhaps they did not want to confront the abomination of grisly personal details. What they didn't know about grandpa's grave couldn't horrify them . . . and the midnight resurrection from a nearby graveyard remained the only available source of cadavers for the medical students around the country.

Periodically, various state legislatures dredged up the matter, usually in response to a local incident that seemed too heinous to be ignored, but they could never muster enough gumption to pass a meaningful bill. Lawmakers could envision only two alternative sources from which they could possibly draw suitable cadavers— executed criminals or unclaimed bodies. Neither held much appeal for their constituents. The former were simply too scarce; the latter were sufficiently numerous but, alone and impoverished as the bodies might have been in life, the lawmakers' constituents wouldn't stomach laws that would foster dismemberment of anyone. As long as the resurrectionists stuck to the potter's field, most ordinary citizens and official agencies were content to look the other way.

Even in the unlikely event of being apprehended, the professional body thief knew that he could expect a token fine or, at worst, a short prison term.

By the late 1870s, the demand for useable cadavers had far outstripped available resources. The professionals sought bodies from any grave, even of prominent citizens like Diedrich Buck, Mary Neidhofer, and Charles Wright in Fort Wayne, but taking the body of John Scott Harrison had gone too far. People demanded official action. In the past, the introduction of legislation to address the issue of anatomical subjects and body snatching always had proved too controversial to succeed. The clamors of the politicians' wealthy constituents and doctors to procure an adequate and legal supply of bodies from among the indigent dead were invariably drowned out by equally vociferous protests from the anti-dissectionists and the advocates for the poor. It therefore became expedient to feign interest in the issue, and then to table any meaningful proposal. Occasionally a watered-down law would pass, generally designed to mollify everyone but satisfying no one. From the New York anatomy act of 1789 to the Ohio bill of 1870, such laws failed to meet the needs of the colleges and only fueled the passion of the anti-dissectionists.

But in 1878, things suddenly were different. Legislators who had borne the public criticism for their past equivocation began to cast off their shrouds of ambivalence to call for immediate legislative reform. They demanded laws that would put teeth into the crime of body snatching but, at the same time, would provide a reliable and adequate source of cadavers for the nation's medical schools. Had they known their local history, they would have recognized the ghostly wails from the Worthington, Ohio, preacher Reverend S.W. Streeter who had demanded much the same reforms from his pulpit forty years earlier.[48] (*See Ch. 6.*)

---

48 Linden F. Edwards, "Body Snatching in 19th Century Ohio," prepared by the staff of the Library of Fort Wayne and Allen County, 1955.

From the roughhewn stage of a fledgling nation, the resurrection drama played out in North America along similar lines as it had in its British counterpart half a century before. But the American curtain dropped in 1878, with John Scott Harrison's naked body hanging in a dark chute of the Medical College of Ohio.

Most colleges of medicine required their students to dissect at least one cadaver with three to five students per body. A year after the infamous Doctors' Riot in New York in 1788, citizens learned about the horrors of mutilation being carried out on stolen corpses. They responded with an angry mob of rioters converging on Broadway for several days, and the state legislature passed an anatomy act. The act, however, was drafted more to prevent the robbing of graves than to provide subjects to the medical colleges. Like its English precedents, the bill provided only the bodies of executed criminals that the court, at its discretion, could compound the death penalty with anatomic dismemberment.

But as had happened in England before, there weren't nearly enough hangings to supply the anatomists. The North American resurrectionists soon followed the practices of their old world predecessors by establishing business arrangements with specific anatomists as new colleges of medicine took root. Even when the more enterprising grave robbers supplied several colleges by shipping the bodies long distances in barrels of whiskey or brine, most states simply ignored the issue as long as possible.

In the Midwest, the anti-dissection movement gained ground. In 1831, the Ohio Assembly made it unlawful to remove a corpse for any purpose, including dissection. Ten years later, only creative politicking and impassioned letters from doctors and enlightened friends prevented the passage of bills that were proposed "to prevent the study of anatomy and surgery" altogether. On March 25, 1870, the Ohio legislature finally managed to pass a law that allowed designated public facilities such as state hospitals and prisons to ship unclaimed bodies to medical schools for dissection.

However, in concession to its anti-dissectionist opponents, they made the process of releasing the bodies so time-consuming that the intervening putrefaction rendered those cadavers useless as anatomic subjects for dissection. The new law only encouraged the state's two most notorious body snatchers, Old Cunny in Cincinnati and Dr. Henri Le Caron in Columbus, to provide subjects, freshly lifted from their graves.

Following the Harrison Horror, the editor of the Cincinnati Daily Gazette proclaimed:

> The law should be changed . . . so as to make the offense [of grave robbing] virtually impossible. Every thinking person will admit that medical colleges must have material for dissection. The welfare of society demands that they should study anatomy from actual dissection. So long as this necessity for subjects exists and there is no legal mode of obtaining a supply, the business of resurrectionists must continue. The responsibility for this outrage rests ultimately upon the legislature.[49]

Even as the state legislature deliberated, the resurrectionists continued their labors. In one night in November 1878, in Zanesville, Ohio, they exhumed four bodies from two separate cemeteries; then were caught after a wild police chase over the countryside. The grave robbers, including a young physician, were fined $1,000 and sentenced to six months in jail, but the governor pardoned them. Although it was clear to everyone that the 1870 law was not working, it took three years to pass an acceptable bill, the Ohio Anatomy Law of 1881. The law called for the delivery of all unclaimed bodies to schools of dissection after twenty-four hours. It made exception for the bodies of "strangers," unless the stranger belonged to the "class, commonly known as tramp."

---

49 Linden F. Edwards, "The Ohio Anatomy Law of 1881, Part III," *The Ohio State Medical Journal* (January 1951), 49–52.

Fort Wayne managed to drag out its body-snatching scandal for nearly a year from the rash of thefts in the fall of 1877 to that winter's arrest of A.E. Van Buskirk and his students and their trials that lasted until the end of May 1878. By then, the Hoosiers had had their fill of the resurrectionists and had begun work on an acceptable statewide anatomy act before the year was out.

The president of board of the Fort Wayne Medical College, the Honorable Joseph K. Edgerton, worked through the Christmas holidays of 1878 to draft the bill that was eventually presented to the Indiana State Assembly. What he did not know was that even as his pen scratched across the page, his physician colleagues from the medical college, Myers and C.B. Stemen, were caught unearthing fresh subjects from the nearby Roanoke, Indiana, cemetery. Edgerton understood the crucial importance of firsthand human dissection for the training of physicians and surgeons, but he had much to learn about what those schools had to do to acquire them. The doctors had claimed that bodies could be purchased in Chicago, and he had no reason to doubt their word.

Edgerton's bill passed the Indiana state legislature in March 1879, but it was similar in intent and content to the 1870 Ohio law. It acknowledged the importance of dissection for the education of doctors and provided that bodies of individuals who died in the custody of the state could be transferred to qualified colleges of medicine. Like the Ohio law, the act required substantial concessions to appease its opponents. The 1879 Indiana act required such Byzantine record keeping of the source and fate of the corpses that, as in Ohio eight years earlier, the cadavers could rarely be released before they had decayed beyond any utility to the medical colleges. But although the Indiana Anatomy Act of 1879 failed to solve the problem entirely, it set the stage for meaningful reform by changing the illegal disinterment of bodies from a misdemeanor to a felony and by acknowledging that some source of legal cadavers needed to be found. In 1904, in response to another body-snatching scandal, that time in Indianapolis, the law was modified to ensure a steady supply of cadavers from among the unclaimed bodies in the state.

By the early twentieth century, scientific advancement began to have its impact on American medical education. Strict academic requirements for admission and graduation applied to every school; the diploma mills closed either voluntarily or in response to the Flexner commission of 1910.[50,51] State anatomy acts by and large had put the resurrectionists out of business for good. Colleges of medicine would, for the foreseeable future, draw their cadavers from the masses of the poor, disconnected, and unwanted. Despite the changes, anatomy had left a stain that would take many years to wash away. By the turn of the century, the professors no longer lurked in the moonlight through the local graveyards. Medical schools no longer opened to a season of resurrection but to the changing colors of autumn leaves. The students received their cadavers through legal channels in a well-scrubbed morgue, but the stigma of dissecting the unclaimed bodies of the poor and forgotten would require most of the century to wash away. The morgue wasn't tucked away in a darkened alley for no reason.

50 A. Flexner, *Medical Education in the United States and Canada* (Washington, DC: Science and Health Publications, Inc., 1910).

51 Thomas P. Duffy, "The Flexner Report—100 Years Later," *Yale Journal of Biology and Medicine* 84 (2011): 269–276.

CHAPTER 16

Blighted School

T HE NEW ANATOMY ACTS successfully shifted the stigma of dissection from the criminal to the poor, but the blemish on everyone involved would take longer to erase. Many of the doctors were content to accept the unseemly practice with its inherent risks of arrest and disgrace as part of learning and doing their business. Big Sommers had simply paid his fine and put the sordid events behind him; others, like the surgeon W.H. Myers, considered a successful snatch as a sort of badge of honor, another notch in his gunstock, regardless of any social or legal repercussions. Myers boasted of exploits like a fisherman with a newly caught trout. Still others, such as the impulsive Professor Clark, fled the state in disgrace. The sensitive demonstrator of anatomy, A.E. Van Buskirk, felt exploited by the sordid business, outraged at the injustice of being convicted of a crime merely because he was doing his job as a teacher of medicine. He surely understood the indignation that ordinary people felt over sepulchral violation of their loved ones, but the anatomist also harbored his own private indignation that people appeared incapable of understanding the importance of proper anatomical study to train competent physicians. In his mind, what he was doing to obtain cadavers was no more or less unseemly whether they came from Chicago or the local graveyard, than dissecting those bodies behind the closed doors of his laboratory. It was the inadequacy of the law that had forced him to deal with criminal body snatchers in order to obtain the subjects that the college required. But it was he, not the real perpetrators, who stood tried, convicted, and humiliated. The stain may have spread widely, but it seeped most deeply within the young demonstrator.

Although the affair had perversely compromised A.E. Van Buskirk, it neither began nor ended with him. Nearly every medical school in the country had been marked by body-snatching scandals, including Columbia, Yale, Maryland, and particularly the Medical College of Ohio where the body of a congressman who was the son of a president had hung naked from a pulley, over a laundry chute. Those schools, however, were sufficiently well established that they could weather the storm and survive, but in Fort Wayne, it was different. The college was too young, untried, and too controversial. The stains were too dark to clear readily. The blight had spread to its roots.

Perhaps those well-meaning men at the Aveline had not planned sufficiently to start their new medical college on a solid footing. After the public meetings in March 1876, the Medical College of Fort Wayne seemed to have had as many adversaries as advocates, but their fervor carried them ahead anyway. Even when shortly after the college had opened and the neighbors had complained about fetid odors emanating from the third floor windows over Wright's Drug Store, each of the founding faculty seemed to have his own personal agenda that went beyond training medical students. Yet the founding doctors had not done enough to garner the support of their colleagues in the growing city, especially among the many physicians who had been left out. Even prior to the medical college, Fort Wayne physicians who were later excluded had prided themselves on being among the finest in the nation, despite evidence to the contrary. Their exclusion still chafed as an intolerable snub.

The Hamilton rape case, at which Myers and Clark had cut ranks with the community physicians, further polarized them from their colleagues. The highly publicized incarceration of Drs. Dills and Buchman cemented the deep resentment between the medical community and its would-be academic physicians. Well before Charles Wright's body had been exhumed, the separate factions of faculty already had held secret meetings to plan the expulsion of their enemies. When the body-snatching scandal broke, the doctors aligned for or against the accused but not always for principles pertinent to the subject of anatomic dissection. Dills and Buchman, released from jail, sided with the demonstrator, going so far as to pay his bail and to testify on his behalf. Their antagonists, Clark and Myers, not only fingered Van Buskirk from the street corner, but testified against him and, thus, against the school and their downtown rivals, Dills and Buchman.

When Squire Ryan remanded the case to the criminal court, the grand jury, in addition to indicting the individual doctors, went so far as to condemn the school as a whole.[52] The newspapers questioned whether or not the beleaguered medical college could survive. The belligerent but powerful Professor Myers must have agreed when he delivered the final blow in the form of his resignation as professor and chief of surgery.

As the scandals had multiplied, both human and financial support for the Medical College of Fort Wayne simply ran dry. Just after commencement ceremonies were held at the Fort Wayne Rink (*see Fig. 11, Ch. 14*) on February 20, 1878, the ill-fated institution closed its doors for the final time. Despite the collective community horror and revulsion toward the college, the graduates appeared, degrees were conferred, and speeches given, without any untoward events. Even the recently resigned professor of surgery, William H. Myers, feigned optimism for the school's future, but he and everyone else knew the organization already lay moribund

---

52 *Fort Wayne Daily News*, January 11, 1878.

upon its own dissection table. In early March, barely two years after the school's founding meeting at the Aveline Hotel, the faculty and board of directors disbanded the college and dissolved its charter well before the demonstrator of anatomy had heard his final verdict.

But despite the cascading events that had doomed the school, many doctors, as well as the city's leading citizens, continued to believe it was advantageous for the city of Fort Wayne to have a medical college. Regardless of their internal disputes, most of the old faculty sympathized with the plight of first-year medical students who were stranded midway through their school tenure. They would need another year in a certified medical college to qualify for their medical degrees.

The school might have officially closed, but the property, the laboratories, the meager equipment, and the offices remained in the hands of the board of directors. For several months prior, Myers and other members of the defunct faculty had been surreptitiously discussing forming a new medical college, one that would ostensibly be more inclusive of Fort Wayne doctors and more responsive to the city at large. Indeed, part of Van Buskirk's defense had been his contention that forming a new medical college under Myers's control had been the crafty old surgeon's goal all along. Thus, almost immediately after the original school closed, doctors and concerned business leaders held meetings to consider establishing a new medical college in Fort Wayne. These conclaves lasted throughout the spring of 1878, even as Judge Lowry attempted to assemble a jury for Van Buskirk's third trial. Whether by personal choice or volitional exclusion, Dr. Van Buskirk disappeared from the rolls of the college and its several new iterations that followed. He likely had had enough of so-called academic medicine for the time being.

The organizers of the new medical college involved a wider spectrum of Fort Wayne's leading citizens who formed a community-based board of directors. The new board then began to recruit new faculty, drawn both from the original academic faculty of the now defunct Medical College of Fort Wayne and from the community of physicians who had not been involved in the old school. First, they needed an unimpeachable dean who would garner and hold the respect of both the doctors and the public. To no one's surprise, the board prevailed upon the distinguished gentleman Dr. Benjamin S. Woodworth, one of Fort Wayne's most admired physicians. Although Dr. Woodworth had been an enthusiastic supporter, after the founding meeting at the Aveline Hotel, he had played only a minor role in the original school's operations. And though he had been, in fact, the treating physician for the ill-fated Charles Wright, Woodworth escaped any aspersions about his implicit involvement with the body snatching.

Dean Woodworth and the board next needed to address the problem of finding an instructor of anatomy, a position that was vital to a successful medical college, but had been so severely tainted by the recent scandals. They must have realized that they could not involve any of the local doctors—neither from the original faculty nor from the community physicians—for such a crucial, yet delicate, position. In light of the ongoing trials, the community would ostracize any local doctor who applied for the job, and from a practical viewpoint, none were qualified. The former professor of anatomy, Harold A. Clark, had left town in disgrace, and his demonstrator, A.E. Van Buskirk, still awaited trial in Judge Lowry's courtroom. As they had before, members of the board, undoubtedly on the advice of the original medical college dean, Dr. Christian Stemen (a prominent local surgeon who had been among the original founders from Cincinnati), turned to their neighbors at the Medical College of Ohio in that city. From there, they recruited the prestigious anatomist, Dr. William H. Gobrecht.

Born in 1828, Gobrecht had served until 1861 as a distinguished professor of anatomy at Jefferson Medical College in Philadelphia. In 1859, he had published a highly respected edition of Erasmus

Wilson's textbook, *A System of Human Anatomy, New and Improved American Edition.*[53] After the Civil War, Gobrecht became professor of anatomy at the Medical College of Ohio in Cincinnati. By hiring him to reassemble and lead an anatomy department in the new school in Fort Wayne, the school would garner immediate experience and unimpeachable national respect, a base upon which the new college could establish the credibility it would desperately need.

Christian Stemen, who had served under Gobrecht in Cincinnati, described the new professor as the most admired anatomist in the country. What he omitted was that, outside of a few academic medical communities, few anatomists could claim to be admired at all.

The board of directors and the new dean then made a concerted effort to involve as many Fort Wayne physicians as possible on the new faculty in order to placate the many critics and skeptics. What their balms could not salve were the deep and festering wounds that continued within the various factions of physicians, especially between the original faculty and those who had been originally excluded. (Membership on the faculty of a college of medicine has always lent a bit of an aura to academic physicians that might, in fact or perception, lend a competitive edge to their medical practices. That perception of qualification perhaps played a more significant role in the nineteenth century than in later times when documentation of medical credentials became routine. However, the conflict between physicians of the gown and of the town continues to develop when they compete for the same patients, reenacting the same farcical drama over and over, without a final act, from the beginnings of university medicine in the nineteenth century to the present day.)

---

53 Erasmus Wilson, *System of Human Anatomy, General and Special.* A new and improved American edition, ed. William H. Gobrecht (Philadelphia: Blanchard and Lea, 1859).

One of the physicians who felt particularly snubbed by his exclusion from the original faculty was Thomas Jefferson Dills, MD, who was one of the first eye, ear, nose, and throat physicians in Fort Wayne. Dr. Dills was best remembered for his refusal to testify in the Hamilton rape case back in November 1877, and for his subsequent conflict with Professor Myers. By the spring of 1878, his court case had advanced all the way to the Indiana Supreme Court, which ruled in his favor, agreeing that physicians should be compensated for their expert testimony. With the formation of the new medical college, all those diversions had ended. The new dean and the board of the new school recognized that they needed a more circumspect view of their new faculty than had previously prevailed, so they invited Dr. Dills as well as his fellow holdout, Dr. Buchman, to join the faculty of the new school. But although Dills and Buchman had been the doctors who had stood by A.E. Van Buskirk and had paid his bail, Buchman's loyalty did not preclude him from taking his old friend's position as demonstrator of anatomy, under Professor Gobrecht, in the new school.

In an attempt to keep the faculty as broadly based as possible and, in fairness, as competent as possible, the new medical school also appointed as professor of surgery the belligerent Dr. William H. Myers who was willing, at least for the time being, to let bygones be bygones.

By May 31, Woodworth had assembled a faculty of seventeen physicians for a new college of medicine. The board of trustees announced the signing of Articles of Association for the school to be named the Fort Wayne Medical College. Those articles granted the board of trustees the power to confer doctor of medicine degrees to all graduates who had completed their first term at the old school, the Medical College of Fort Wayne.

That same day, in a different venue, the jury found the former demonstrator of anatomy from the defunct school, Dr. Aaron E. Van Buskirk, guilty of the misdemeanor of body snatching. That time it was not Dr. Buchman but another colleague, Mr. H.C. Hartman, who covered A.E.'s expenses, including a fine of $400 and $150 in court expenses. After all, A.E.'s position at the old college had already been filled in the new one, by his previous benefactor, Alpheus Buchman.

Despite the politick of its new founders, the newly formed Fort Wayne Medical College proved even more tenuous than its predecessor and lasted only one year. Just as the first school had been too exclusive, Dr. Woodworth and his board of directors, in their attempts to garner support, could have been a bit more selective with their faculty appointments. Perhaps the old doctor, in his attempt to pacify everyone, had not been sufficiently attentive to the political, fiscal, and legal realities of running a college of medicine. The faculty may have been new, but it was comprised of old combatants whose swords were had been sheathed but not shelved.

The important participants, the business leaders Edgerton and McCulloch, and the doctors Stemen, Woodworth, and even Myers, must have foreseen that the Fort Wayne Medical College was, from its hasty beginning, already irrevocably crippled beyond its capacity for rehabilitation. Perhaps they knew that the new school could only initiate a halting step toward some final resolution. Many of them also might have felt an obligation to the matriculated students to provide a means for them to complete their training. Medical colleges, including the old and new iterations in Fort Wayne, generally required successful completion of two terms over two years to qualify for graduation with the degree of doctor of medicine. The term ran from September to February. Many of the former students did stay with the new Fort Wayne Medical College; they received their degree in the spring of 1879. However, those select students who were in a position to predict firsthand the tenuous nature of the of the foundling college, did not remain. The sons of prominent faculty, despite their fathers' ostensible support of the new college, sought more established educational institutions in distant cities. Herschel Myers transferred to his father's alma mater in Philadelphia and received his MD degree from Jefferson Medical College. Norman Teal, who was professor of orthopedics, sent his son to Rush Medical College in Chicago.

The exact details of what happened within the halls of the Remmel Building on Broadway and Washington during the 1878–79 academic year have not survived, but old battle lines clearly remained. William H. Gobrecht's popular lectures on anatomy could not dispel ongoing dissension that swirled through the hallways like the autumn leaves on Broadway Street outside. For the most part, the college-based faculty who had been with the school from the beginning, many of whom had been recruited from Cincinnati, opposed the community practitioners who had fought their way onto the faculty of the new school. The registrar, C.B. Stemen, one of the original founders at the Aveline in 1876, began to make his presence felt. The board of trustees had had their fill of squabbling doctors, but they listened to the academic core, Drs. Stemen and Gobrecht. By the end of the term, the academics, including newcomer Gobrecht, had had enough. The issues within the Fort Wayne Medical College may have been different on the surface, but the unresolved internal struggles among the physicians made the school's future untenable. To compound the misery, the school was on the brink of financial collapse.

In August 1879, the board of trustees announced that they were unable to raise sufficient funds to continue to carry the project forward. Again, they abandoned the school.

Those community-based physicians, Dills, Buchman, their old antagonist Myers, and Myers's brother-in-law, Hiram Van Sweringen, retained the space in the raw old building and its fixtures on Broadway and tried to hang on. They formed a third iteration of a medical college using the original title, The Medical College of Fort Wayne, with T.J. Dills as dean, but they had lost their more academic core including the influential Christian Stemen and the nationally prestigious William H. Gobrecht.

Meanwhile, many of the original founders of the college who had gathered at the Aveline three years earlier were unwilling to allow their dream of a sustainable medical college in Fort Wayne to go unfulfilled. They reassembled a board of trustees and recruited the prestigious Hugh McCulloch, who had been secretary of the treasury under both presidents Lincoln and Johnson, and who was president of the Indiana State Bank. With McCulloch's blessing and the use of the McCulloch mansion in which to house it, they founded yet another, the fourth, medical college with many of the old faculty and many of the same members of the original board.

On August 22, 1879, the new institution was incorporated in the state of Indiana as the Fort Wayne College of Medicine. It would reside in the McCulloch mansion on Calhoun Street (*see Fig. 12*), just a few blocks from its rival, the upstart Medical College of Fort Wayne, which had remained in the old building at Broadway and Washington. The prestigious anatomist Professor Gobrecht agreed to serve as dean for the new college for its first year, with his former student and colleague C.B. Stemen as registrar. Gobrecht returned to Ohio three years later, by which time the Fort Wayne College of Medicine was well established and seemed destined to sustain itself for the foreseeable future.

Thus, between 1879 and 1882, Fort Wayne could "boast" of not one, but two colleges of medicine. They competed tooth and nail. They fought both privately and publicly over which was the legitimate successor to the original and which the interloper.

In the spring of 1880, the Medical College of Fort Wayne's announcement of their "sixth" fall term drew the scorn of their rival Fort Wayne College of Medicine with a long, seven-point essay from the Fort Wayne College of Medicine's registrar, Dr. Stemen, who disputed the very existence of the Medical College of Fort

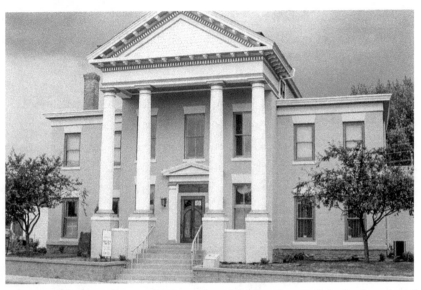

Figure 12. The McCulloch mansion in 2001. This was the site of the final version of the Fort Wayne College of Medicine. Photographed by the author.

Wayne and its successors.[54] Dr. Stemen pointed out that, at best, the school had only been in existence for one year and thus had no claim on the alumni of the old colleges dating to 1876.

Both schools coveted the loyalty of the Fort Wayne practicing physicians, but some flavor of academic legitimacy would loom more crucial. Although the schools needed referrals from area physicians to sustain their institutions' financial futures, a gathering public demand for some type of academic credentialing for colleges of medicine became the more urgent issue.

Around the same time that the original college (Medical College of Fort Wayne) was founded in 1876, representatives of twenty-two American medical colleges had met in Philadelphia to form the American Association of Medical Colleges. (That organization continues to oversee and provide credentialing of schools of medicine today.) The newly formed agency had approved the first iteration of the Medical College of Fort Wayne, but the

---

54 *Fort Wayne Gazette*, February 18, 1880.

approval was dropped with the closure of the school in 1878, and it was never renewed. By 1880, the association recognized the Fort Wayne College of Medicine, but not its rival. Without the needed accreditation, the school could not carry on. The Medical College of Fort Wayne, the first and third iterations of medical schools in Fort Wayne, closed its doors on Broadway and Washington for the final time in 1883. The fixtures were sold to the only available buyer, its competitor for the previous four years, the Fort Wayne College of Medicine, for the sum of $50. By that time, the faculty was undoubtedly glad to be rid of their obligation even for such a paltry sum.

By 1885, the surviving Fort Wayne College of Medicine listed seventeen faculty members and seven "assistants." Christian Stemen, the sole representative of the original founders, served as dean. Drs. Rosenthal and Myers were conspicuous in their absence, apparently content in private practice. Dr. A.E. Van Buskirk, Stemen's old student, had returned to academia as professor of surgical anatomy. The school persisted for another twenty-nine years until 1905 when it merged with several other Hoosier-propriety medical colleges to form the Purdue University Medical School. The Purdue school eventually merged with Indiana University to form the contemporary Indiana University School of Medicine.

The old combatants of Fort Wayne seem to have put down their arms for the college's final years prior to the mergers. (*See Fig. 13.*) The final announcement lists thirty-nine faculty among whom were the dean, Christian Stemen; William H. Myers; Myers's brother-in-law, Hiram Van Sweringen; and Alpheus Buchman. The professor of surgical anatomy, A.E. Van Buskirk, had died the previous year, but his nephew, E.M. Van Buskirk, MD (the author's grandfather and namesake), who had graduated in 1902, then served on the faculty. Dean Christian Stemen remained for its final year before becoming a trustee of Purdue University.

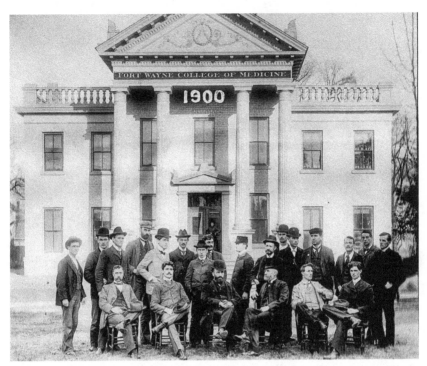

Figure 13. The Fort Wayne College of Medicine, 1900. A.E Van Buskirk, MD, professor of surgical anatomy is seated in the first row, third from the right, with a gray-white beard and wearing a top hat. E.M. Van Buskirk is a first year student, standing in the center, wearing a flat top cap. Like his uncle, he is shown in profile. From the Van Buskirk Family Archive.

CHAPTER 17

Bessie's Gift

ESSIE VAN BUSKIRK was correct when she assured her nephew, my father, that "they rang the courthouse bells" to announce her father's innocence in 1878, twelve years before she was born. What she might not have known was that those bells had rung for her father's acquittal in the Wright trial, but not for his succeeding conviction for the Buck resurrection. Nor did Bessie seem to know that after his acquittal for Wright, A.E. had been promptly arrested, and ultimately tried and convicted for stealing Diedrich Buck's body.

The story of the notorious body snatcher lay deeply embedded in my family lore as a mysterious, abstract, but intriguing yarn from the murky past. My mother loved the mysterious romance of the tale as an ironic anecdote rather than a serious part of family history. She often thrilled us with embellished tales of our relative having been tarred and feathered, driven out of town "on a rail to Deadwood, South Dakota."

One day I found an old leather medical kit in our attic: It was engraved with the initials "A.E. Van Buskirk, MD." I carefully opened the dry and cracked leather to reveal some long expired medications in little stoppered tubes and a few yellowed business cards. (*See Figs. 14 & 15.*)

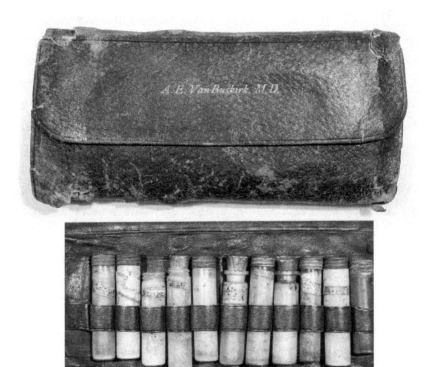

Figure 14. A.E. Van Buskirk's Traveling Medical Kit.

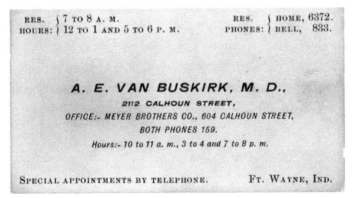

Figure 15. The business card of A.E. Van Buskirk, MD. From the Van Buskirk Family Archive.

The cards were engraved with an address and office hours, and noted "special appointments by telephone." On inquiring, I learned that these objects had belonged to the famous (or infamous) grave robber of our family lore. With such official-looking impedimenta as well as a formal photograph of the distinguished gentleman that is engraved *A.E. Van Buskirk, M.D., Surgical Anatomy (see Fig. 16)*, it was hard to imagine him tarred and feathered and driven out of town. But it was enough of a mystery to stimulate me as a young man to want to determine what had really happened. In the waning years of my own father's life, he, too, sometimes seemed unclear about the details, on one occasion even declaring, "He never did it, you know!"

After her older sister, Minnie, died in 1956, Bessie sold her house and boarded with another elderly woman (though younger than she was), where she remained until the mid-1980s. In 1987, deep into her tenth decade of life, alone and with no family left in Fort Wayne, Bessie was living in The Lawton Nursing Home, near Lawton Park in Fort Wayne. Only after my father had died, while my daughter Sarah and I were conducting research for this book, did we learn from the Lawton staff that her nephew, my father, sometimes visited Bessie in the nursing home. Some dozen years previously, while my father was writing a historical article about the old medical colleges in Fort Wayne, they had begun discussing the 1877 body-snatching episodes.[55] He had written to ask her for any recollections she might have had of her father, A.E. When they discussed his notorious case, she always began by saying, "Oh, it all happened before my time . . ." It was clearly a subject on which the ninety-year-old woman did not like to dwell.

---

55 Edmund L. Van Buskirk, "The Fort Wayne Medical Schools 1876–1905 and the Union with Purdue University," *Indiana Medical History Quarterly*, Indiana Historical Society (February 1976): 3(1): 55–66.

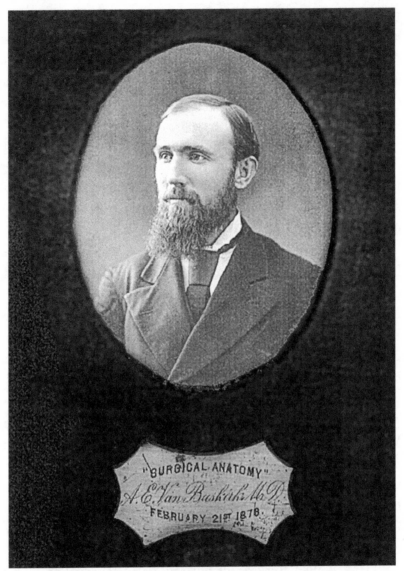

Figure 16. A.E. Van Buskirk, MD, professor of surgical anatomy, February 21, 1878. From the Van Buskirk Family Archive.

However, between a local historian recounting the story, or the local newspapers periodically dredging up the ghoulish details for a Sunday feature article, the topic was difficult to avoid. In 1973, Fred J. Reynolds, the aforementioned historian, relayed the grisly events to the members of the Fort Wayne Quest Club in a presentation entitled "Anatomical Materials." On October 28, 1990, just two months before Bessie died, the *Fort Wayne News Sentinel* featured an article entitled "Thieves in the Night," that depicted the hideous details even naming her father as the "City doctor (who) preyed upon graves."[56]

The story in our family thus ebbed and flowed between A.E.'s outright innocence to his being tarred and feathered and run out of town. As Bessie would say, it had actually all happened long before she was born; the details were bound to have become repressed or exaggerated over time.

Regardless of Bessie's recollections, what we now know is that before 1878, the main sources of anatomic "subjects" for medical colleges had been the local graveyards, and that in Fort Wayne, it had been A.E. Van Buskirk's job to obtain those "subjects." We also know that most of the "snatches" went unnoticed. Even in the face of compelling, if circumstantial, evidence to the contrary, A.E. had been acquitted of stealing the body of Charles Wright, but he also was convicted of stealing the Diedrich Buck body. By the time of A.E.'s final conviction in May 1878, the Medical College of Fort Wayne had long dissolved even as a new iteration was in the offing. A.E. and Mary Jane Van Buskirk dropped off the records for a while, perhaps to spend the summer in eastern Ohio where they had a farm near Mary Jane's family. They returned to Fort Wayne in time for the birth of their first child, Minnie Belle, who was born on October 17, 1878.

Dr. A.E. Van Buskirk sat out the era of the dueling medical colleges in Fort Wayne; he probably had had enough of squabbling doctors to last a lifetime. He resumed his private practice of medicine in Fort Wayne with an office first in his home at 12 Locust Street and later near their home at 244 South Calhoun Street, where they remained until 1881. However, around that time, Mary Jane seems

---

56 Alan Derringer, "Thieves in the Night," *Fort Wayne News Sentinel*, October 28, 1990.

to have gone back to Ohio, at least temporarily, while, for next three years, A.E. lived in a local boarding place known as The Harmon House. Perhaps his wife needed to come out from under the shadow of the grisly trial that still loomed over them, or she wanted to escape the epidemic fevers that were sweeping the city at that time. A.E., however, undoubtedly stayed behind to maintain the medical practice he had worked so hard to restore.

During that period, A.E. and Mary Jane had two more children, both born in Fort Wayne: their second child, Etta May, was born on June 22, 1881; their third, Robert Jaye, on August 17, 1883. By the mid-1880s, A.E. had established a reputation as a dedicated practicing physician in the city. The local newspapers seem to have forgotten the scandals that had graced their papers a decade earlier. They now extolled Dr. Van Buskirk on South Calhoun Street who labored to save other sick children while his own were dying at home.

Sadly, despite any precautions they may have taken, the family had not been able to escape the pestilence pervading the city. Little Robert died of scarlet fever on December 19, 1885, followed a few weeks later by his sister Etta May. The grief-stricken parents had two more children, Bertha May, who died in infancy, and Harry Franklin, who died at the age of two, on June 16, 1889.

Their sixth and youngest child, Bessie Louella, was born the following year on May 3, 1890, in Fort Wayne. A few years later, A.E. and Mary Jane bought a lovely Victorian-style home a bit farther up the block at 416 South Calhoun where they had plenty of street-front office space for A.E. When the city of Fort Wayne renumbered the street addresses in 1904, their address at number 416 became 2112 South Calhoun Street. The house remained in the family for nearly half a century, lapsing in and out of family occupancy over the years. (*See Fig. 17.*)

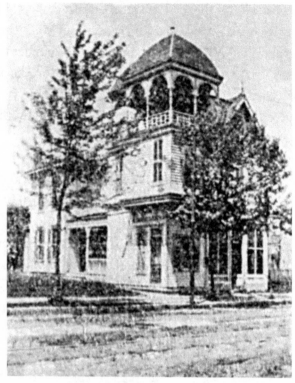

Figure 17. The home and office of A.E. Van Buskirk and family at 2112 S. Calhoun Street, Fort Wayne. Photo from the Van Buskirk Family Archive.

As her father had been portrayed in his obituary, Bessie, too, had seemed destined for a hard life. The death of four of her older siblings before she was born hung like a morbid pall over her family. Her mother appeared to be chronically ill, perhaps downtrodden by her husband's early disgrace and the loss of her young children. As a teenage girl, Bessie attended A.E.'s Saturday morning lectures at the medical college, instilling in her a dream that, one day, she too could become a physician. Her father's early death put a sudden end to whatever dreams Bessie might have had along those lines: A.E. had left them their house but little financial security.

There seemed to be no question that Bessie would need to learn a skill that would support herself and her mother. Thus, she enrolled at the International Business College of Fort Wayne from which she graduated in 1906, at the age of 16. (*See Fig. 18.*) The International Business College taught penmanship, typewriting, and shorthand, vital skills for modern business. Now eminently employable at the age of 16, Bessie supported her mother until she died in 1919.

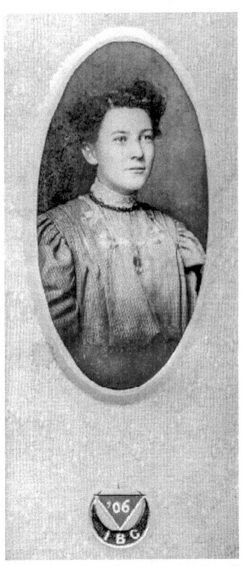

Figure 18. Bessie Van Buskirk, age 16. International Business College. Photo from the Van Buskirk Family Archive.

Bessie, however, did not pursue any of those specific business skills that she had learned, but rather became a dressmaker, working out of her house. It was fortuitous that she had developed her dressmaking proficiency early because it sustained her for most of her life. She listed herself as a dressmaker in the Fort Wayne city business directory and, in later years, in the telephone directory well into the mid-1960s.

After her father died, Bessie and her mother remained in the house at 2112 South Calhoun St. with Bessie earning a modicum of income from dressmaking. Clearly, their financial situation was precarious at best for there was little in A.E.'s estate—a bit of medical equipment and about $800 of accounts receivable. Mary Jane applied successfully to be declared exempt from estate tax.

The older sister, Minnie Belle, had, in 1902, married a man named Gustav Woebbeking, a mercurial man, vacillating from job to job, place to place. He had worked as a molder for the railroads but seemed to change jobs every year or so, from molder to grocery clerk to traveling salesman. In 1903, Minnie gave birth to a stillborn child, and they had no more children.

Around 1907, Bessie and her mother, Mary Jane, temporarily moved in with Minnie and Gustav on Wall Street, next door to the grocery store where Gustav was then working. Their mother entered into an agreement with a man named Michael Bohan for him to use the South Calhoun property until Mary Jane regained it with a quitclaim deed for $1 in 1919.[57]

In 1910, Bessie and Mary Jane relocated again; by 1911, they had disappeared from Fort Wayne and Allen County records. It is most likely that Bessie and her mother had moved east to Ohio, near Mary Jane's Gray family. In 1918, they are listed in Akron, Ohio, sharing an apartment on Fay Street where Bessie, by then just 28 years of age, continued to take in sewing work. However,

---

57 Similar to a promised intention of a handshake, a quitclaim deed transfers title to property without either an extensive title search or a guarantee of the owner's title.

Mary Jane, who had been in poor health since A.E.'s death, became mortally ill, and in 1919, they returned to Fort Wayne, where she died of stomach cancer that March. The death certificate describes a chronic stomach ulcer as a contributory factor, which could have been the underlying cause of Mary Jane's chronic malaise. After a brief stay with Minnie and Gustav, Bessie returned to her father's old house on South Calhoun Street that they'd regained from Mr. Bohan a few years earlier.

Meanwhile, Bessie's older sister Minnie's husband, Gustav Woebbeking, continued to shift from one occupation to another, which included being a fishmonger, traveling salesman, and salesman for the Gunder Agency during the 1920s. In 1924, Gustav and Minnie gave up their own home and moved back into the old family home on South Calhoun with Bessie, but that only lasted a few years. Gustav's restlessness persisted. In 1929, he went to work in his brother Christian's restaurant and moved out of the house, leaving Minnie with Bessie. Gustav boarded alone in a house on W. Washington Boulevard, but he suffered a heart attack and died on Dec 26, 1932.

Minnie Belle and Bessie lived together in Fort Wayne, first in their parent's old home on Calhoun Street. Bessie later revealed that Minnie had suffered chronically poor health all of her life, and that it fell to Bessie to care for her. In 1941, they sold the old family home and lived in a variety of smaller places until buying a house at 921 Cottage Avenue in 1950. Bessie continued to work as a dressmaker throughout the 1940s and 1950s, apparently as their primary source of income. Bessie had written that she'd cared for her sick sister since her mother had died, living and working as a sort of resident nurse and seamstress until Minnie died in 1956.

Twenty years later, in 1975, Bessie reminisced in a letter to my father that she was glad she had sold her house and then boarded with another woman. She pointed out that, in her room at the boarding house, it was the first time in her life that she was independent and free to do as she pleased. She noted that she was writing to him on a Christmas morning, enjoying the snow, and being glad that it was her landlady's task to shovel it from the walks. She was relishing the night before when she had attended a midnight Mass and returned home in the wee hours of the morning. Perhaps referring to her squelched dream of being a doctor in a family of doctors, Bessie reiterated that, although not a doctor, she had spent her whole life caring for the sick, first her mother and then her sister. (*See Fig. 19.*)

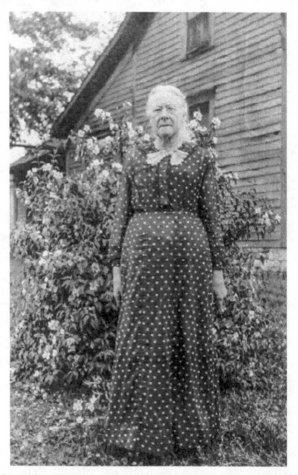

Figure 19. Bessie Van Buskirk, on her own in Fort Wayne, ca. 1965. Photo from the Van Buskirk Family Archive.

But Bessie's freedom came too late, for as she entered the nonagenarian years, she realized that her days of independence were, of necessity, drawing to a close. In 1987, Bessie moved into the Lawton Nursing Home where she died on December 14, 1990 at the age of 100. The previous year someone had taken her picture in the church parking lot on Mother's Day. They had given her flowers because she had been the oldest one there. (*See Fig. 20.*)

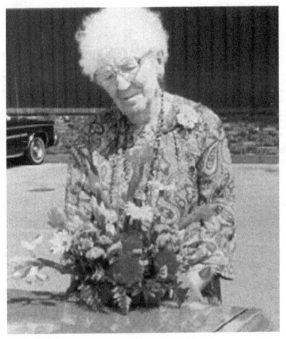

Figure 20. Bessie Van Buskirk, age 99, 1989. Photo from the Van Buskirk Family Archive.

Some eight years later, when my daughter Sarah and I were gathering information about our infamous body snatching– physician relative, we visited his grave in the Lindenwood Cemetery. We couldn't ignore the irony of his tomb lying for all eternity only a stone's throw from the now defunct and unmarked gravesite of Charles Wright. Sitting in a row were the stones of A.E. Van Buskirk, his wife, Mary Jane, and their spinster daughter,

Bessie, on a gradual slope and mounted just above a poignant line of four little stones that commemorated the toddlers who had died in the pestilence of the 1880s. I noted that the stone for Bessie, in the same rose-colored granite as the monuments of her parents, lacked an inscription of the date of death. (*See Fig. 21.*)

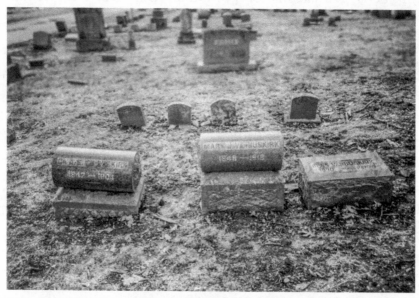

Figure 21. The gravesite of members of the A.E. Van Buskirk family in Lindenwood Cemetery, Fort Wayne, Indiana. Front row, left to right: A.E., Mary Jane, and Bessie. The four small stones in the background are those of four children who died young. Photographed by the author.

I learned from the cemetery office that they had received the cremated remains of Bessie Van Buskirk from Indiana University School of Medicine. There appeared to be no remaining relatives, so the urn had been buried under the stone without a date of death—so I had it inscribed. Of greater curiosity to me was the revelation that, in her final years, Bessie Van Buskirk, daughter of a man who had been accused of arranging resurrections, had arranged for her own body to be donated to the Indiana University School of Medicine to undergo anatomical dissection.

It is tempting to postulate that she had done so as a gesture to make amends for her father's role in acquiring anatomical subjects for the old medical college; it is a possible explanation, given her frequent reference to those events that had so affected her father's life as well as her own. On the other hand, I suspect that she was well aware of the new anatomy acts passed in the mid-twentieth century that discouraged or prohibited the use of unclaimed bodies for anatomic dissection. By the 1980s, most states had instituted body donation programs as the primary, if not exclusive, source of cadavers. In the latter decades of the twentieth century, posthumous organ and body donation became a well-accepted, publicly encouraged, humanitarian act.

As Bessie continued to protest the injustice of it all, she would ask, "How were the students to learn?" Aside from her recriminations over her father's activities, I believe it is equally likely that she decided to address the issue in the only way she knew. Whether done in recompense for her father's deeds or simply as an altruistic act of a lonely woman, Bessie Louella Van Buskirk, spinster, who had spent her life caring for her sick mother and sister, had voluntarily donated her body for anatomic dissection.

As Bessie had wished and anticipated, her shriveled body had lain supine upon the dissection laboratory's stainless steel table, inanimately submitting to the ministrations of uncertain hands. Regardless of her reasons for being there, she had known as well as anyone what would transpire on that table. She must have been confident that her decision would allow the hands that gradually stripped her tissues away to become more and more adept as the months passed, and that one day they would manifest the sensitive hands of the physician palpating an offending tumor or the sure hands of the surgeon removing it. Had Bessie still been aware, she would have thought that those hundred years had all been worthwhile.

Afterword

Y THE EARLY YEARS of the twenty-first century, most contemporary medical schools had substantially reduced the amount of time that their students devoted to firsthand cadaveric dissection. Moreover, the quantity of dissection varies widely among the various schools from virtually none to a nearly complete dissection. In lieu of a full direct cadaveric experience, anatomy laboratories typically substitute prosected specimens, three-dimensional digital imagery, and plastinated models. An overview of these processes is as follows:

- Prosected specimens are dissection regions, such as an arm or a chest that has been previously prepared by faculty or senior student prosectors for demonstration to anatomy students.

- Three-dimension modeling is derived from computer software that is continuously updated and finessed

- Plastination involves replacing water and lipids in a fresh cadaver with a plastic solution that allows the specimen to retain many of it original properties indefinitely.

Recently, however, medical students who had not been exposed to cadaveric dissection began to suspect a deficiency in preparation for their first exposure to clinical medicine. The curricula of nearly all

US medical schools now include some direct exposure to cadavers but the amount continues to vary widely.

Some critics refer to cadaveric dissection as an unnecessary, arcane ritual, a procedure akin to an initiation rite into the society of physicians and surgeons. Newer methods of cadaver preservation and simulation undoubtedly expedite and facilitate the teaching of gross anatomy. On the other hand, Bessie Van Buskirk would have been the first to explain that there is more to learn from dissection than the cadaver's gross anatomy. Of the many arguments for and against cadaveric dissection, I believe Jeanette Der Bedrosian, a writer for *Johns Hopkins Magazine* expressed it best:

> One week into med school, they are handed their first patient. He'll teach them more about gross anatomy than they ever thought they could absorb in seven weeks. But he'll also teach them how to care. How to detach. How to work as a team. A sense of curiosity and discovery. How to navigate the emotions they'll face when they become fond of a patient but have to put him through the most painful experience of his life in order to make him well again.[58]

The firsthand exposure to the anatomy of the human body in all its detail has always been an immensely practical matter of adding a multifaceted keystone to the foundation of a physician's training—a passage yes, but much more than a ritual.

---

58 Jeanette Der Bedrosian, "First-Year Medical Students Still Rely on Cadavers to Learn Anatomy," *Johns Hopkins Magazine*, Winter 2016.

Bibliography

Adams, George W. *Doctors in Blue*. Baton Rouge, LA: Louisiana State University Press, 1952.

Ball, James Moores. *The Body Snatchers*. 3rd ed. New York: Dorset Press, 1989. (Originally published in 1928.)

Bartholow, Roberts. *A Practical Treatise on Materia Medica and Therapeutics*. 5th ed. New York: D. Appleton and Company, 1884.

Bierce, Ambrose. *The Devil's Dictionary*, 1911 edition (Cornell University Library, 2009).

Cooper, Astley. *The Lancet*. 1:1–8. Surgical Lecture, 1824.

Der Bedrosian, Jeanette. "First-Year Medical Students Still Rely on Cadavers to Learn Anatomy." *Johns Hopkins Magazine*, Winter 2016.

Derringer, Alan. "Thieves in the Night." *Fort Wayne News Sentinel*, October 28, 1990.

Doyle, Arthur C. *The Return of Sherlock Holmes*. London: Georges Newnes, Ltd., 1905.

Duffy, Thomas P. "The Flexner Report—100 Years Later." *Yale Journal of Biology and Medicine*, 2011.

Edgar, William S., ed. *St Louis Medical and Surgical Journal*. 11 (September 1874): 485.

Edwards, Linden F. "Body Snatching in 19th Century Ohio." Prepared by the staff of the Library of Fort Wayne and Allen County, 1955.

— "The Ohio Anatomy Law of 1881, Part III." *The Ohio State Medical Journal*, January 1951.

— "Cincinnati's 'Old Cunny.' A Purveyor of Human Flesh." Prepared by the staff of the Public Library of Fort Wayne and Allen County. 1955.

Feltoe, Charles Lett. *Memorials of John Flint South.* London: John Murray, Albemarle Street, 1884.

Fitzharris, Lindsey. *The Butchering Art: Joseph Lister's Quest to Transform the Grisly World of Victorian Medicine.* New York: Scientific American / Farrar, Straus, and Giroux, 2017.

Flexner, A. *Medical Education in the United States and Canada.* Washington, DC: Science and Health Publications, Inc., 1910.

Fort Wayne Daily News. November 24, 1877.

— November 26, 1877.

— November 27, 1877.

— December 13, 1877.

— December 27, 1877.

— January 11, 1878.

— January 23, 1878.

— January 28, 1878.

— February 6, 1878.

Fort Wayne Daily Sentinel. "Esculapian Enterprise." March 15, 1876.

— November 28, 1877.

— November 29, 1877.

— January 28, 1878.

Fort Wayne Gazette. February 18, 1880.

Fort Wayne Weekly Sentinel. June 9, 1875.

Geison, Gerald L., ed. *Physiology in the American Context, 1850–1940.* New York: Springer, 1987.

Gray, Henry. *Anatomy: Descriptive and Surgical.* London: John W. Parker and Son, 1858.

Holy Bible. OT. Num. 19:11–22.

Hutton, Fiona. *The Study of Anatomy in Britain, 1700–1900.* London and New York: Routledge, 2015.

Juettner, Otto. *Daniel Drake and his Followers.* Cincinnati: Harvey Publishing Company, 1909.

Ludmerer, Kenneth M. *Learning to Heal.* New York: Basic Books, Inc., 1985.

New York Times. "Medical Schools Show First Signs of Healing from Taliban Abuse." Jan. 15, 2001.

Nuland, Sherwin B. *Leonardo da Vinci*. New York: Viking, 2000.

Saunders, J.B. deC.M. and O'Malley, Charles D. *The Illustrations from the Works of Andreas Vesalius of Brussels*. Cleveland: World Publishing Co., 1950.

Shultz, Suzanne M. *Body Snatching: The Robbing of Graves for the Education of Physicians in Early Nineteenth Century America*. Jefferson, North Carolina and London: McFarland and Company, 2005.

Sievers, Harry J. "The Harrison Horror." Prepared by the staff of the Public Library of Fort Wayne and Allen County. 1956.

Singer, Charles. *The Evolution of Anatomy*. New York: Alfred A. Knopf, 1926.

Taylor, John H. *Death and the Afterlife in Ancient Egypt*. Chicago: The University of Chicago Press, 2001.

Van Buskirk, Edmund L. "The Fort Wayne Medical Schools 1876–1905 and the Union with Purdue University." *Indiana Medical History Quarterly*. Indiana Historical Society. February 1976.

Van Buskirk, E.M. *The Van Buskirks of Indiana*. Amherst, MA: Genealogy House, 2018.

Williams, P.L.; Warwick, R.; Dyson, M.; and Bannister, L.H. *Gray's Anatomy*. 37th ed. New York: Churchill Livingstone, 1989.

Wilson, Erasmus. *System of Human Anatomy, General and Special*. A new and improved American ed. Edited by William H. Gobrecht. Philadelphia: Blanchard and Lea, 1859.

Acknowledgements

ROM A FOURTH GENERATION PHYSICIAN, this was a project of deep exploration into arcane, seemingly trivial, events of late 19th century medicine that permeated our family lore for a hundred years. For the most part, it amused and tantalized but for some, it rubbed an open sore that needed the healing balm of verifiable data about what really happened.

Such data comes only from reliable sources such as the many city, county and state historical societies who, on my behalf, sought obscure records of forgotten people and events that played a role in my story. In particular, I thank the Allen County-Fort Wayne Historical Society and the Indiana State Historical Society for providing original photographs, with permission to reproduce them, for many of the illustrations herein. I also have profound respect for the many anonymous librarians who play such a crucial role in projects of this nature. I especially thank the Allen County Public Library in Fort Wayne, Indiana for hosting our long hours of research and retrieving seemingly lost sources of information.

For helping bring this three decade old project to fruition, I am grateful to Linda Roghaar, Publisher, White River Press. I am also indebted to her staff: Jean Stone for her patient and meticulous copy editing, Doug Lufkin for design, and Janet Blowney for proofreading.

From my tiny home office, I could not produce a work like this without the love and unmitigated support from my wife, Bette. Her infinite patience, rereading multiple drafts and her allowing my books and files to occupy far more than their allotted space in our condominium made my progress smooth and comfortable.

About the Author

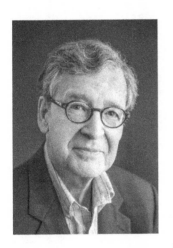

E. Michael Van Buskirk, born in Lafayette, Indiana in 1941, received bachelor and master degrees from Harvard University and a Doctor of Medicine from Boston University in 1968. Dr. Van Buskirk retired in 2004 from a distinguished academic career in ophthalmology with some 200 publications including four books about glaucoma. He founded and edited the *Journal of Glaucoma*. Among Dr. Van Buskirk's numerous awards and honorary lectureships over five continents were the Fankhouser Medal from the University of Basel and that of Distinguished Alumnus from the Department of Ophthalmology, Harvard Medical School.

His first non-medical book was a genealogically oriented tale of Van Buskirks in the settlement of North America. *Daughter, Doctor, Resurrectionist*, the author's second book written for a general readership, also finds its roots in family lore.

CPSIA information can be obtained
at www.ICGtesting.com
Printed in the USA
FFHW020901291019
55841780-61713FF